Rhinoplasty

McGraw-Hill Plastic Surgery Atlas

Peter J. Taub, MD, FACS, FAAP
Professor, Surgery and Pediatrics
Associate Program Director
Division of Plastic and Reconstructive Surgery
Mount Sinai Medical Center and Kravis Children's Hospital
Director, Craniomaxillofacial Surgery
Co-Director, Mount Sinai Cleft & Craniofacial Center
New York, New York

Stephen B. Baker, MD, DDS, FACS
Program Director and Associate Professor
Department of Plastic Surgery
Georgetown University Hospital
Washington, DC

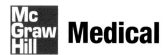

New York Chicago San Francisco Lisbon London Madrid Mexico City
Milan New Delhi San Juan Seoul Singapore Sydney Toronto

Rhinoplasty: McGraw-Hill Plastic Surgery Atlas

1 2 3 4 5 6 7 8 9 0   CTP/CTP   15 14 13 12 11

ISBN 978-0-07-159049-5
MHID 0-07-159049-8

This book was set in Sabon by Thomson Digital.
The editors were Brian Belval and Cindy Yoo.
The production supervisor was Sherri Souffrance.
The illustration manager was Armen Ovsepyan; the illustrator was Kip Carter.
Project management was provided by Aakriti Kathuria, Thomson Digital.
The designer was Eve Siegel; the cover designer was Anthony Landi.
China Translation & Printing, Ltd. was the printer and binder.

This book is printed on acid-free paper.

Library of Congress Cataloging-in-Publication Data
Taub, Peter J.
  Rhinoplasty : McGraw-Hill plastic surgery atlas / Peter J. Taub,
Stephen B. Baker.
      p. ; cm.
  Includes bibliographical references and index.
  ISBN-13: 978-0-07-159049-5 (hardcover : alk. paper)
  ISBN-10: 0-07-159049-8 (hardcover : alk. paper)
  I. Baker, Stephen B. II. Title.
  [DNLM: 1. Rhinoplasty—Atlases. WV 17]
  LC classification not assigned
  617.5'230592—dc23
                                              2011031209

McGraw-Hill books are available at special quantity discounts to use as premiums and sales promotions, or for use in corporate training programs. To contact a representative please e-mail us at bulksales@mcgraw-hill.com.

*To my many mentors over the years, most notably
Dr. Kawamoto who taught me much of what went into this text
and gave me the inspiration to discover the rest.*
Peter J. Taub

*To my family, Margie and Stephen, for their endless love, laughter, and support.
To my patients who have entrusted me with their care, allowing me to grow as a surgeon.
To my residents who challenge me and add mirth to the journey.*
Stephen B. Baker

Contents

Contributor

Jay Meisner, MD, FACS
Clinical Assistant Professor, Surgery
Mount Sinai Medical Center
Chief, Plastic and Reconstructive Surgery
Bronx Veteran's Administration Hospital
New York, New York
Coding

Preface

Rhinoplasty is one of the most challenging endeavors a surgeon can undertake. It is one of a handful of procedures that requires an abundance of experience to learn and a career to master. The various anatomical components are interrelated and manipulation of one area has predictable effects on one or more other components. The various surgical techniques can alter not only form but also function. A superb aesthetic result means little if there is compromise of normal nasal function. Even a brief exposure to rhinoplasty will highlight the patients' high expectations. As such, the surgeon's expectations should be even higher. Within the field of rhinoplasty surgery, there are a limitless number of possible maneuvers and interventions, which is only mastered by a thorough understanding of anatomy and pathology in addition to a well-thought-out treatment plan.

The following text and illustrations are a cumulative effort of surgeons and artists designed to provide the most relevant information in the clearest format. It is not designed to encompass all there is to know about rhinoplasty, but rather to form the stepping-off point from which students, residents, and surgeons should begin their understanding of the procedure. It is organized into sections that address the relevant anatomy, operative setup, surgical steps, and important practical information related to patient care and reimbursement.

During the interview process, the surgeon should develop a complete understanding of the patient's concerns, decide if these are real or imagined, devise a well-thought-out treatment plan, and be confident that he or she can carry out the plan. The present text serves as a well-illustrated guide to the common concerns with which most patients present. It is organized by anatomic location and covers in detail the numerous maneuvers that are frequently used to shape the various parts of the nose. As techniques continue to evolve, the newer methods should be incorporated continuously with the well-established ones described herein.

It should follow that the need for revision following primary rhinoplasty is to be expected on occasion. All surgeons have complications. The nationally reported rate of revision following primary rhinoplasty ranges from 8% to 15%.[1,2] Logically, the incidence will be higher earlier in one's career but should diminish with time, experience, and most of all critical review of one's results. Experienced surgeons who perform revision surgery often achieve a high level of satisfaction among their patients. Still, complications can occur despite technically well-performed surgery. The surgeon who undertakes either his or her own or another's revision should specifically understand the primary surgical alterations and have a plan of how to achieve definite improvement.

Peter J. Taub, MD, FACS, FAAP
Stephen B. Baker, MD, DDS, FACS

REFERENCES

1. Rees TD. Postoperative considerations and complications. In: Rees TD, ed. *Aesthetic Plastic Surgery*. Philadelphia, PA: WB Saunders; 1980.
2. McKinney P, Cook JQ. A critical evaluation of 200 rhinoplasties. *Ann Plast Surg*. 1981;7:357–361.

Rhinoplasty

Chapter 1. Nasal Anatomy: Bony Support

- The osseous framework of the nose is composed of two semi-rectangular and obliquely oriented nasal bones that extend approximately one-third of the length of the nasal dorsum (Figures 1-1 and 1-2). As the strongest substance in the nose, the bony vault provides support and stability.
- In adults, the mean length of the nasal bones is approximately 20 mm. They are widest in the region of the nasofrontal suture—approximately 14 mm and narrowest at the nasofrontal angle—approximately 10 mm. The thickest portion is superiorly near the nasofrontal suture, where it averages 6 mm and is thinnest inferiorly.
- Osteotomies should be designed to cut through intermediate or transition zones of bone thickness. The region from the piriform to the radix along the nasal process of the maxilla has been shown to be no more than 2.5 mm thick and can be predictably osteotomized with small osteotomes.[1]
- Each nasal bone articulates with four other bones in the face: the frontal bone superiorly, the ethmoid bone superolaterally, the maxilla laterally along the piriform aperture, and the contralateral nasal bone medially. The lateral articulation between the nasal bone and the maxilla is not truly within the valley between the nose and malar complex, but rather extends onto the nasal sidewall. What is referred to as an osteotomy of the nasal bones actually traverses the nasal process of the maxilla. The superior extent of each bone is dense and serrated and forms a narrow articulation with a notch in the frontal bone. By contrast, the inferior border is thin but supported from beneath by overlapping attachments with the paired upper lateral cartilages. The lateral border is perhaps the most important since it is in this region that the bones commonly fracture and controlled osteotomies are performed. Here, the bone is similarly serrated. Along the superior portion, it is beveled such that the edge faces inwards, while inferiorly the converse is true. The medial border articulates with the contralateral nasal bone and, as it approaches the frontal bone, becomes thicker than it is below.
- Caudally, the edges of the nasal bones overlie the cranial extent of the paired upper lateral cartilages. Similarly, the midline septum begins outside the bony pyramid but continues beneath it proximally.
- The external surface of each bone begins as a concave structure and becomes convex inferiorly. It is also convex from medial to lateral. The topography of the inner surface is the opposite of the external surface and thus, convex superiorly, concave inferiorly, and concave from side to side.
- Each of the nasal bones is covered by the *procerus* and *compressor naris* muscles.
- Each nasal bone is perforated in the center by a foramen, which carries a small venous tributary.
- The lacrimal bone lies posterior to the articulation of the nasal bone and the maxilla. It is the smallest and most fragile bone of the face and is situated in the anterior portion of the orbit.
  - It articulates with four bones, including the frontal and ethmoid bones, the maxilla, and the inferior nasal concha. The lateral surface of the bone, which faces the orbit, is divided by the posterior lacrimal crest into an anterior portion and a posterior portion.
  - Anterior to the crest lies the lacrimal sulcus, which unites with the frontal process of the maxilla. The upper part of this fossa contains the lacrimal sac, while the lower part contains the nasolacrimal duct.
    - This is relevant since osteotomies of the nose traverse the nasal process of the maxilla and can be injured if the osteotomy is placed too far posterior. The medial surface, which faces the nose, possesses a longitudinal furrow, which corresponds to the lateral crest. The area anterior to the furrow forms part of the middle meatus of the nose, and the area posterior articulates with the ethmoid.

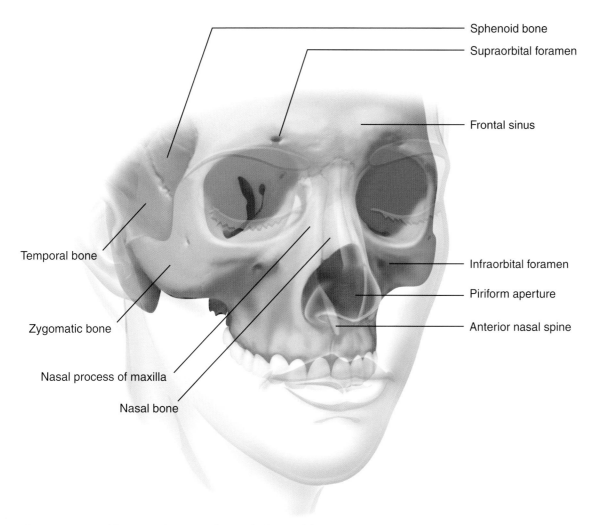

Sphenoid bone

Supraorbital foramen

Frontal sinus

Temporal bone

Infraorbital foramen

Piriform aperture

Zygomatic bone

Anterior nasal spine

Nasal process of maxilla

Nasal bone

Figure 1-1. Facial bones as they articulate with the nasal bones.

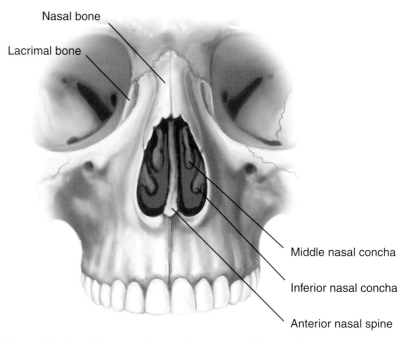

Nasal bone

Lacrimal bone

Middle nasal concha

Inferior nasal concha

Anterior nasal spine

Figure 1-2. Nasal bones and internal structures of the nasal cavity.

- The nasal conchae, or turbinates, are shelves of bone, which extend from the lateral nasal sidewalls and curl within the air passages (Figures 1-2 and 1-3). They serve to direct inspired air into a steady, regular flow across the surface mucosa. The mucosa is composed of pseudostratified ciliated cells.
  - The inferior turbinates are the largest turbinates and are responsible for the majority of airflow deflection, humidification, heating, and filtering. The bulk of inhaled airflow travels between the inferior and the middle turbinates.
  - The middle turbinates are almost as long as the inferior turbinates but do not come as far anterior. The middle turbinates cover the openings of the maxillary and ethmoid sinuses. They serve to protect the sinuses from direct contact with pressurized nasal airflow.
  - The superior turbinates are smaller structures, which protect the olfactory bulb. They shield the nerve axons piercing through the cribriform plate into the nose.
  - All three turbinates are innervated by pain and temperature receptors, via the trigeminal nerve (CN V).

REFERENCE

1. Harshbarger R, Sullivan PK. Lateral nasal osteotomies: Implications of bony thickness on fracture patterns. *Ann Plast Surg*. 1999;42:365.

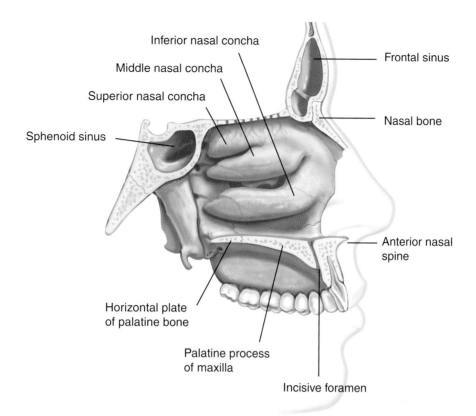

Figure 1-3. Internal topography of the lateral nasal cavity.

Chapter 2. Framework: Cartilaginous Support

- The cartilaginous framework of the nose is composed of paired upper and lower lateral cartilages that extend out from the end of the bony pyramid. Each pair of cartilages has a distinctly different shape (Figure 2-1).
- The upper lateral cartilages are relatively flat and form the caudal sidewalls of the nasal pyramid. The medial border of each lies against the septum in the midline. The lateral border rests near the piriform aperture within the sidewalls of the nose. Their angle with the midline septum forms the internal nasal valve.
- The lower lateral cartilages have a more intricate structure. They are curved strips that bend around the alar rims and function to maintain competence at the external nasal valve (Figure 2-2). Each is composed of three parts, or crura.
  - The medial crura approximate each other at the midline within the substance of the columella.
  - The middle crura rest within the nasal tip. The angle between the medial and middle crura is roughly 20% to 25%.
  - The lateral crura are relatively flat compared to the middle and medial portions. They flare out within the substance of the columella. The two nasal domes are separated from each other by 3 mm to 4 mm and an angle of 70 degrees to 80 degrees. From the lateral genu, the lateral crura generally parallel the alar rims along the anterior third. They then diverge posteriorly at a 30- to 45-degree angle.[1]

- There are several ways in which the upper cartilages attach to their lower counterparts. Most commonly, the caudal edges of the upper cartilages form a scroll or clasped-hands connection with the cephalic edges of the lower cartilages. The two edges may also simply adjoin one another and rarely, they may overlap one another.[1]
- The midline cartilaginous septum divides the interior of the nose into two vestibules (Figure 2-3). It is composed of hyaline cartilage anteriorly and bone inferiorly and posteriorly. It forms a central structure onto which the superior border of the upper lateral cartilages rest. Beneath the septum lies the vomer, while posteriorly it joins the perpendicular plate of the ethmoid. Its caudal margin has a defined posterior septal angle, a middle septal angle, and an anterior septal angle. These angles are important in the definition of the nasal tip.
- Smaller sesamoid cartilages and dense fibrous tissue lie between the lateral crus and the piriform aperture.

REFERENCE

1. Daniel RK. The nasal tip: Anatomy and aesthetics. *Plast Reconstr Surg*. 1992;89:216.

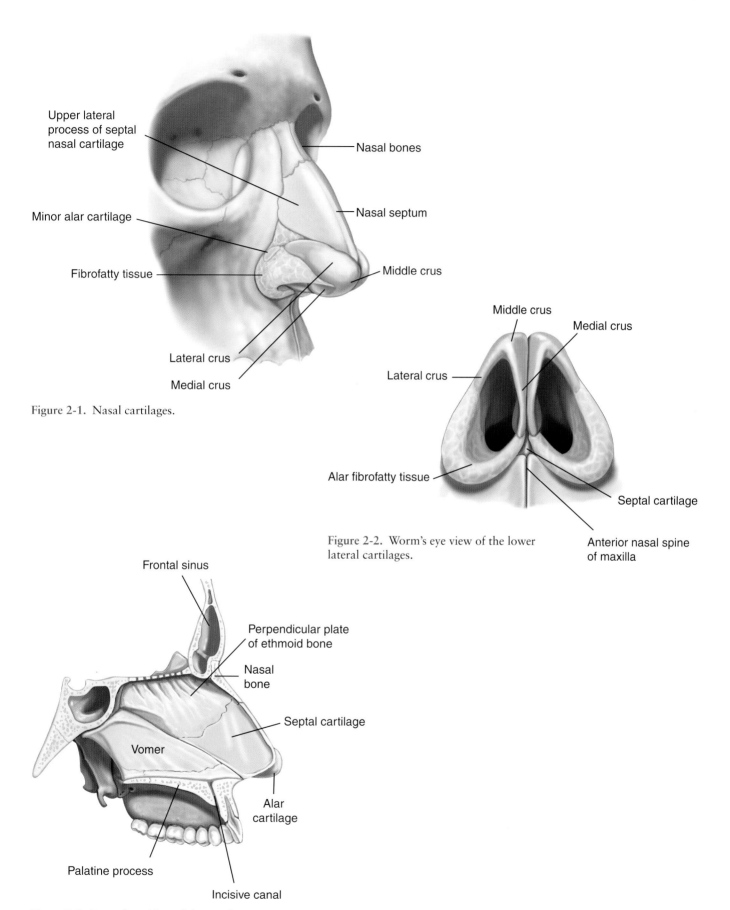

Upper lateral process of septal nasal cartilage

Nasal bones

Minor alar cartilage

Nasal septum

Fibrofatty tissue

Middle crus

Lateral crus

Medial crus

Figure 2-1. Nasal cartilages.

Middle crus

Medial crus

Lateral crus

Alar fibrofatty tissue

Septal cartilage

Anterior nasal spine of maxilla

Figure 2-2. Worm's eye view of the lower lateral cartilages.

Frontal sinus

Perpendicular plate of ethmoid bone

Nasal bone

Septal cartilage

Vomer

Alar cartilage

Palatine process

Incisive canal

Figure 2-3. Lateral position of the nasal septum.

Chapter 3. Vascularity: Arterial Supply

- The vascular supply and lymphatics of the nose are found superficial to the musculature. Dissection during rhinoplasty in the proper areolar tissue plane below the muscles preserves blood supply to the periphery and minimizes postoperative ecchymosis and swelling.
- Externally, the anterior ethmoidal artery and the superior labial artery, as well as nasal branches from the infraorbital artery and the angular branch of the facial artery provide vascularity to the nose (Figure 3-1). The infraorbital branch of the internal maxillary artery and the ophthalmic branches of the internal carotid system supply the more dorsal regions.
- The lateral nasal artery is a branch of the angular artery and is considered the most important contributor to the cutaneous blood supply of the nasal tip. This artery is located 2 mm to 3 mm above the alar groove. If an alar base excision is to be performed in an open rhinoplasty, it is important to make sure the incision does not extend beyond the alar groove.[1]
- Internally, the vascular supply of the medial and lateral walls of the nasal cavity (Figures 3-2 and 3-3) arises from several arterial systems:
  - The anterior ethmoidal artery arises from the ophthalmic artery of the internal carotid system and divides into medial (septal) and lateral branches to supply the nasal cavity. Along with the posterior ethmoidal artery, it supplies predominantly the superior portions of the lateral vestibule.
  - Similarly, the posterior ethmoidal artery arises from the ophthalmic artery of the internal carotid system and divides into the medial (septal) and lateral posterior nasal arteries.
  - The sphenopalatine artery arises from the maxillary artery of the external carotid and also divides into medial (septal) and lateral branches. It supplies predominantly the posterior and inferior portions of the septum and lateral vestibule, respectively.
  - The greater palatine artery arises from the maxillary artery of the external carotid. It travels to the anterior lower part of the nasal septum via the incisive foramen of the hard palate.
  - The superior labial artery arises from the facial artery of the external carotid system. It supplies predominantly the anterior portions of the vestibule.[2] All five arterial systems that supply the septum meet in a watershed area, in the anterior portion of the septum called "Kiesselbach plexus."
- A submucosal plexus deep to the nasal mucosa drains into the sphenopalatine, facial, and ophthalmic veins, providing venous drainage from the internal portions of the nose. Externally, the blood drains to the facial vein via its angular and lateral nasal tributaries.
- The venous plexus serves an important role in the body's regulation of heat. Air is warmed as it enters the nose and heat is exchanged to the environment.
- One important note is that the veins in the nose communicate with the cavernous sinus of the central nervous system via valveless conduits. Thus, there is the potential for nasal infection to ascend to the brain and meninges.
- Lymphatics in the nose drain the superficial mucosa posteriorly to lymph nodes in the retropharynx and anteriorly to the submandibular or deep cervical nodes in the neck.

REFERENCES

1. Bafaqeeh SA, Al-Qattan MM. Simultaneous open rhinoplasty and alar base excision: Is there a problem with the blood supply of the nasal tip and columellar skin? *Plast Reconstr Surg.* 2000;105:344.
2. Hollinshead W, Rosse C. *Textbook of Anatomy.* 4th ed. Philadelphia, PA: Harper and Row; 1985:980–981.

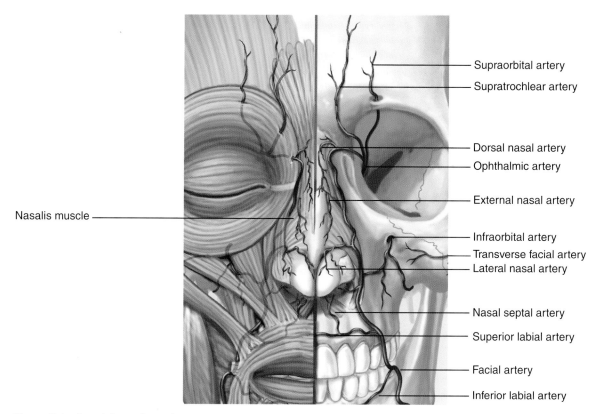

Supraorbital artery
Supratrochlear artery
Dorsal nasal artery
Ophthalmic artery
External nasal artery
Infraorbital artery
Transverse facial artery
Lateral nasal artery
Nasal septal artery
Superior labial artery
Facial artery
Inferior labial artery

Nasalis muscle

Figure 3-1. Arterial supply to the nose.

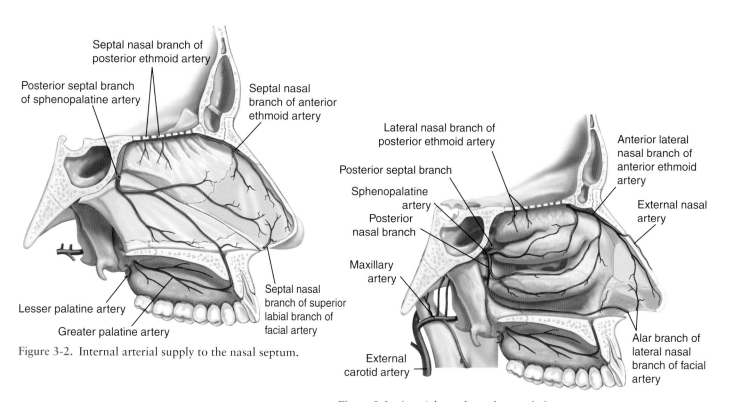

Septal nasal branch of posterior ethmoid artery
Posterior septal branch of sphenopalatine artery
Septal nasal branch of anterior ethmoid artery
Lesser palatine artery
Greater palatine artery
Septal nasal branch of superior labial branch of facial artery

Figure 3-2. Internal arterial supply to the nasal septum.

Lateral nasal branch of posterior ethmoid artery
Posterior septal branch
Sphenopalatine artery
Posterior nasal branch
Maxillary artery
External carotid artery
Anterior lateral nasal branch of anterior ethmoid artery
External nasal artery
Alar branch of lateral nasal branch of facial artery

Figure 3-3. Arterial supply to the conchal system.

Chapter 4. Innervation of the Nose

- Innervation of the nasal mucosa can be divided along an oblique line, running from posterior superior to anterior inferior.
  - The anterosuperior mucosa is predominantly supplied by the ophthalmic nerve, the first division of trigeminal nerve (CN V), via anterior and posterior ethmoidal nerves.
  - The posteroinferior mucosa is predominantly supplied by the maxillary nerve, the second division of the trigeminal nerve (CN V), via the nasopalatine nerve medially and the greater palatine nerve laterally.
- Externally the dorsum is supplied by the ophthalmic division of the trigeminal nerve, via the infratrochlear nerve and a branch of the anterior ethmoidal nerve (Figure 4-1).
- The anterior ethmoidal nerve, a branch of the nasociliary nerve, travels vertically within a groove on the internal surface to provide sensation to the lateral nasal vestibule.

- The external alae are innervated via branches of the infraorbital nerve off the maxillary division of the trigeminal nerve.
- Smell is transmitted via olfactory nerves, which run within the superior portions of the septum and lateral walls of the vestibule (Figures 4-2 and 4-3). The individual nerves pass through the cribriform plate along the floor of the anterior fossa.[1,2]

REFERENCES

1. Hollinshead W, Rosse C. *Textbook of Anatomy.* 4th ed. Philadelphia, PA: Harper and Row; 1985:980–981.
2. Hollinshead WH. *Anatomy for Surgeons: The Head and Neck.* 3rd ed. Philadelphia, PA: J.B. Lippincott Company; 1982:245–248.

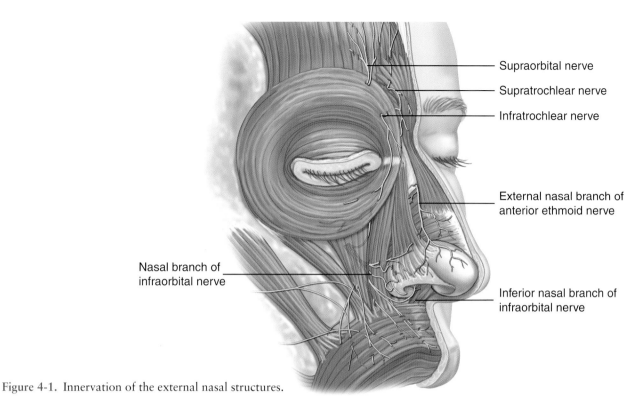

Supraorbital nerve

Supratrochlear nerve

Infratrochlear nerve

External nasal branch of anterior ethmoid nerve

Nasal branch of infraorbital nerve

Inferior nasal branch of infraorbital nerve

Figure 4-1. Innervation of the external nasal structures.

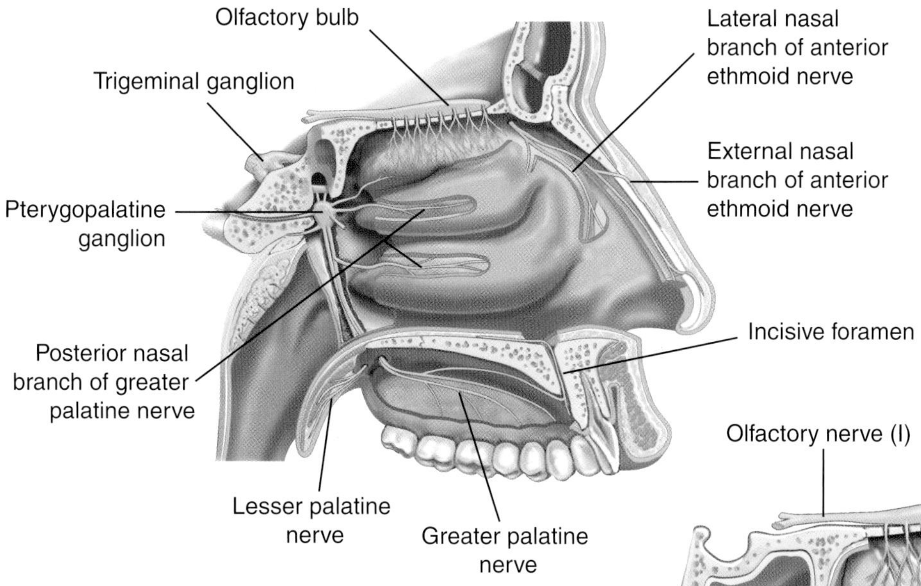

Olfactory bulb

Trigeminal ganglion

Lateral nasal branch of anterior ethmoid nerve

External nasal branch of anterior ethmoid nerve

Pterygopalatine ganglion

Incisive foramen

Posterior nasal branch of greater palatine nerve

Lesser palatine nerve

Greater palatine nerve

Figure 4-2. Innervation to the conchal septum.

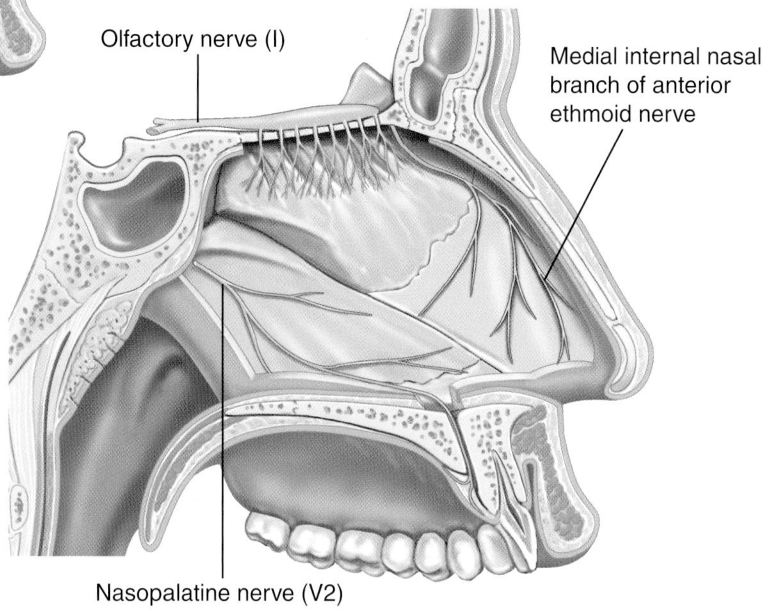

Olfactory nerve (I)

Medial internal nasal branch of anterior ethmoid nerve

Nasopalatine nerve (V2)

Figure 4-3. Innervation to the nasal septum.

Chapter 5. Muscles of the Nose

- The musculature of the nose may be broadly divided by function into elevators, depressors, compressors, and dilators (Figure 5-1).
- The *procerus*, an elevator, is a small pyramidal muscle that lies deep to the superior orbital artery and nerve. The procerus arises from the fascia covering the lower part of the nasal bones and upper part of the lateral nasal cartilage, inserts into the skin over the lower part of the forehead between the two eyebrows (the fibers of the procerus decussate with those of the *frontalis*), and functions to pull the skin between the eyebrows inferiorly assisting in flaring the nares.[1]
- The *levator labii alaeque nasi* arises from the frontal process of the maxilla alongside the nose. Part of this muscle inserts into the nasal skin and the upper edge of the lower lateral cartilage, but the majority passes obliquely downward to the skin and muscle of the upper lip. The nasal portion of this muscle serves to widen the nares, and the labial portion serves to depress the nasal tip.[1,2]
- The *nasalis* is a sphincter-like muscle that originates from the maxilla near the canine fossa and divides into two portions: an alar portion and a transverse portion (Figure 5-2).
  - The alar portion goes to the nostril and enters the skin across the rear circumference of the lateral crus. It functions to expand the nostril across its alar portion.
  - The transverse portion of this muscle goes upward to insert on the upper edge of the upper lateral cartilage and the lower edge of the nasal bone. It acts to compress the nose across its transverse portion.
- The *depressor septi* is a small, paired muscle located on either side of the nasal septum. It runs between the buccal mucosa and musculature of the upper lip. Some patients with depressor muscle hyperactivity will complain about drooping of the nasal tip, elevation and shortening of the upper lip, and increased exposure of the maxillary gums when smiling. An "overactive" *depressor septi* muscle that contributes to drooping of the nasal tip is diagnosed by the "smile test" (ie, the nasal tip drops slightly when the patient smiles). Division of this muscle has been described as a treatment for the patient with a positive smile test.[3]
- The only dilator of note is the *dilator naris*. Its anterior portion originates on the alar cartilage and inserts in the skin near the margin of the nostril. Its posterior portion is beneath the *quadratus labii superioris* muscle. It also originates from the alar cartilages as well as the margin of the nasal notch of the maxilla and it inserts in the skin near the margin of the nostril.
- The *orbicularis oris* originates on the maxilla and mandible, inserts in the skin encircling the lips, and functions to purse the lips.

REFERENCES

1. Figallo E, Acosta J. Nose muscular dynamics: The tip trigonum. *Plast Reconstr Surg.* 2001;108(5):1118–1126.
2. Hollinshead WH. *Anatomy for Surgeons: The Head and Neck.* 3rd ed. Philadelphia: J.B. Lippincott Company; 1982:296–297.
3. Rohrich RJ, Huynh B, Muzzaffar AR, et al. Importance of the depressor septi nasi muscle in rhinoplasty: Anatomic study and clinical application. *Plast Reconstr Surg.* 2000;105:376.

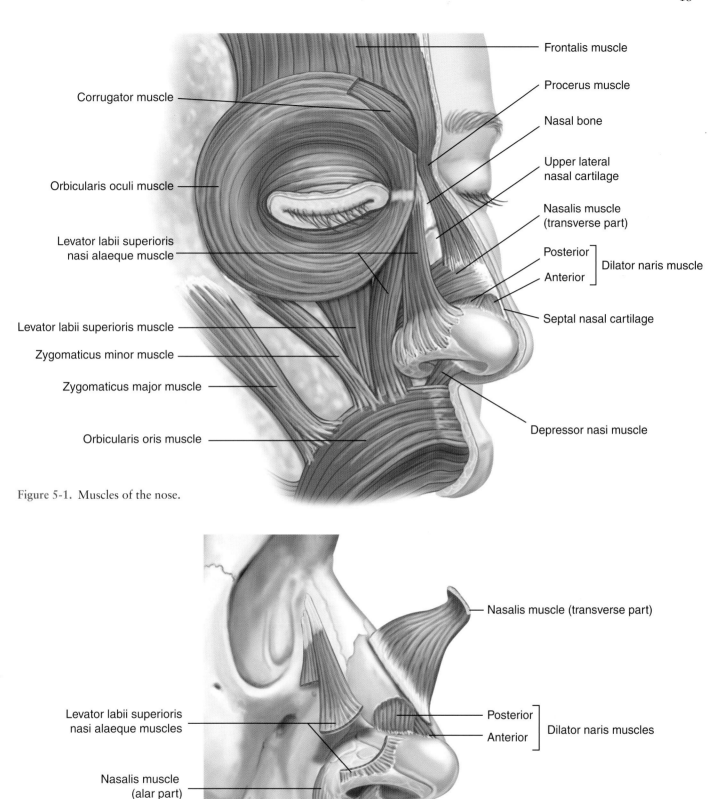

Frontalis muscle

Procerus muscle

Nasal bone

Upper lateral
nasal cartilage

Nasalis muscle
(transverse part)

Posterior ⎤
⎥ Dilator naris muscle
Anterior ⎦

Septal nasal cartilage

Depressor nasi muscle

Corrugator muscle

Orbicularis oculi muscle

Levator labii superioris
nasi alaeque muscle

Levator labii superioris muscle

Zygomaticus minor muscle

Zygomaticus major muscle

Orbicularis oris muscle

Figure 5-1. Muscles of the nose.

Nasalis muscle (transverse part)

Posterior ⎤
⎥ Dilator naris muscles
Anterior ⎦

Levator labii superioris
nasi alaeque muscles

Nasalis muscle
(alar part)

Nasalis muscle
(transverse part)

Depressor septi nasi muscle

Figure 5-2. Deeper muscles of the nose with certain muscles reflected.

Chapter 6. Treatment Planning: Facial Aesthetics

THE INTERVIEW

- The preoperative, and often repeat, consultation is critical to the success of rhinoplasty surgery. Numerous important points need to be addressed by the surgeon in consultation. A patient's motivation for surgery is of utmost importance. What is the reason the patient is interested in surgery? Is the patient undergoing the procedure for self image or in response to external pressures? It is important that the patient is internally motivated to undergo rhinoplasty surgery, with its inherent risks and complications, and is not feeling pressure from another person. It is also important that the patient is not doing it to regain a lost romance or be rehired to a lost job.

- Historically, authors and artists have depicted the "normal" face in various ways. With regards to the nose, its structure has been described in both absolute and relative lengths, widths, and angles. In reality, there is no true normal nose but values and relationships exist that are considered normal for most persons. Rather than subjecting each prospective patient to a plethora of measurements, the surgeon should be familiar with the important ones and decide which are most useful. After facial analysis, any deviations from normal should be discussed with the patient to discuss the patient's level of motivation for treatment. In almost all cases, the patient's desires should take precedence over the surgeon's effort to meet established "norms" in rhinoplasty surgery. Rhinoplasty requires an aesthetic eye as well as a sharp pencil.[1]

- The surgeon should identify functional problems as well aesthetic concerns and prioritize these in a problem list. It is important to educate the patient about any factors that may make a result fall short of the planned goals and set realistic expectations for surgery.

- It is important to question the patient about any functional problems when planning the operative steps.
  - Is there a history of difficulty breathing?
  - If so, is this seasonal or sporadic?
  - What medications does the patient take and how frequently?

- Several maneuvers performed in rhinoplasty can actually lead to airway obstruction. In these cases, counteractive procedures need to be incorporated into the treatment plan and the patient needs to be counseled about the possibility of new or persistent airway obstruction. In situations where aesthetic goals (ie, narrowing of the nose) may be limited due to functional concerns, it is preferable to err on the side of function rather than create airway problems while attempting to achieve aesthetic goals.

- In order to successfully meet the patient's goals, it is important that the patient clearly communicate the desired changes that are to be achieved. Occasionally, a patient will offer a broad concern such as "I just don't like my nose." In this case, the surgeon may be able to identify aspects of the nose that deviate from the aesthetic norm. When these features are tactfully presented to the patient, there is frequently immediate agreement and a clarification of treatment objectives. The surgeon should feel that he is not leading the patient. To some extent, the result depends on the anatomy and physiology with which the patient presents. It is important that the patient realizes the limitations to what can be achieved in given individuals.

- Similarly, the surgeon must be able to identify the areas of concern. One of the most crucial aspects of the rhinoplasty consultation is to make certain that the surgeon understands the patient's goals and that these goals are realistic. Computer imaging is a useful tool to help determine patient goals and will be discussed in this chapter. The surgeon must also honestly assess his ability to achieve the result. It is wise to be conservative in rhinoplasty surgery at the beginning of one's career. This may mean referring a difficult case to a more experienced surgeon or staying within one's comfort zone to avoid doing irreparable harm. It is better to return for a minor revision than create the need for a major revision.

THE EXAMINATION

- The six standard preoperative rhinoplasty views are frontal (Figure 6-1), oblique (Figures 6-2 and 6-4), and lateral (Figures 6-3 and 6-5) as well as worm's eye (Figure 6-6).

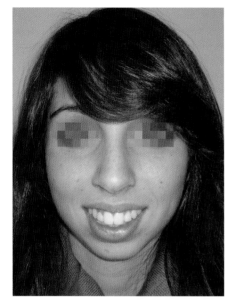

Figure 6-1

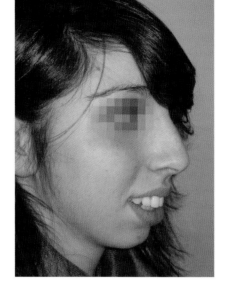

Figure 6-2

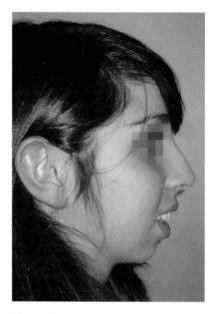

Figure 6-3

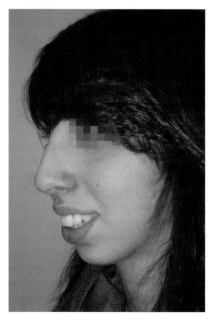

Figure 6-4

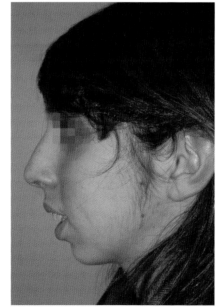

Figure 6-5

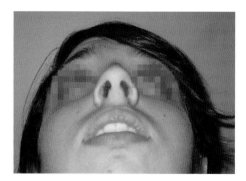

Figure 6-6

- Numerous findings on a patient's physical exam may pose limitations to the expected outcome irrespective of the skill of the surgeon. Despite the artistry with which the supportive bone and cartilage are manipulated, the ultimate aesthetic outcome of the nose is based on how the overlying skin drapes over the supporting framework. Thick and thin skin can both predispose to suboptimal outcomes. Thick skin draped over even the most well-crafted bone and cartilage will hide the detail in these supporting structures. In contrast, thin skin is unforgiving in that all imperfections can be visible. Suture knots, as well as minor irregularities, can become alarmingly apparent requiring revision surgery.

- **Frontal view**: From the patient's frontal view, several important landmarks and relationships should be identified.

  - *Facial dimensions*: The face may be divided into various parts as a means of evaluating areas of imbalance. Vertically, the distance from a horizontal line across the hairline to a line across the eyebrows defines the upper third of the face. The middle facial third is the distance from a line between the eyebrows to the subnasale and the lower facial third from the subnasale to the bottom of the chin. Although these have traditionally been defined as facial thirds, the lower third is slighter larger than the middle third, and the middle third is slightly longer than the upper third.[2,3] Horizontally, equal fifths can be created by lines running vertically through the lateral and medial canthi of each eye.

  - *Alar width*: The width of the nose at the alar base should approximate the span between the medial canthi (Figure 6-7). Wide alar bases may require skin and/or soft tissue excision.

  - *Nasal width*: The width of the nose at the level of the nasal bones as well as the alar base should be evaluated. In general, the width of the nasal bones at their base should be four-fifths of the width of the alar base. Wide nasal bones may require osteotomy and infracture.

  - *Dorsal aesthetic lines*: As important as any component of the nasal evaluation, the surgeon must note the appearance of the dorsal aesthetic lines (Figure 6-8). By definition, they originate on the supraorbital ridges near the medial end of the eyebrow and begin to converge along the glabellar area. They are narrowest at the level of the medial canthal ligaments and then diverge gradually to end at the tip-defining points.

  - *Nasal tip*: The appearance of the tip should be evaluated in isolation and as it relates to the nasal dorsum. The tip-defining points are an important landmark in tip analysis and occur at the transition point between the medial and lateral crura of the lower lateral cartilages. In photographs, the tip-defining points are identified as two bright spots that reflect an external light source. Tip projection, position and the distance between the highlights, the angle of divergence between the crura, and the length of the middle and lateral crura should also be evaluated. The thickness of the nasal skin and the strength of each section of alar cartilage are assessed by visualization and palpation. Tip projection and rotation are best evaluated on the lateral view. The nasal tip is perhaps the most defining feature of a nose. In one random series, the tip-defining points were 8.9 +/- 1.6 mm separate from each other.[4] The course of the lateral crura of the lower lateral cartilages should be noted. In some patients, the lateral crura diverge from the rim at an angle greater than the normal 30 to 45 degrees. This anatomic variation produces a round tip often described as a "parentheses" deformity on frontal view.[5] Aside from the aesthetic implications, the malposition of the lateral crura places them at risk for injury when making a standard intracartilaginous incision.[6] The "boxy tip" is due to an increased angle of divergence between the genu of the lower lateral cartilages (more than 30 degrees), a widened domal arc (more than 4 mm), or a combination of the two.[7]

  - Hyperactivity of the *depressor septi nasi* muscle has been noted to contribute to drooping of the nasal tip. This may be diagnosed preoperatively by observing the patient at rest and then when smiling. Muscle contraction will worsen the deformity and provide an indication to address this paired muscle at surgery.[8]

  - *Nasal deviation*: The degree of nasal deviation must be assessed in every rhinoplasty patient. Several points can be used to denote nasal midline: midglabella, mid-dorsum, nasal tip, central cupid's bow depression, maxillary dental midline, and chin midline. In almost every patient, these points are not on a straight, vertical line. It is imperative to inform the patient of these deviations preoperatively. This is especially important in the patient with subtle facial asymmetry who complains of a deviated nose but is unaware of their underlying facial asymmetry. These patients will complain of nasal deviation yet when the lower half of the nose is covered and the upper half of the nose is related to the upper facial midline marks, it looks on the midline. However, when the upper half of the nose is concealed, and the lower half of the nose is compared to lower facial midline, it appears symmetric. In these patients the midline of the nose is following the asymmetry of the face, and it will be impossible to make the nose straight without compromising facial aesthetics.

- **Lateral view**: On the lateral view, the landmarks should include the glabella, radix (nasion), nasofrontal angle, supratip, tip-defining points, infratip lobule, columella,

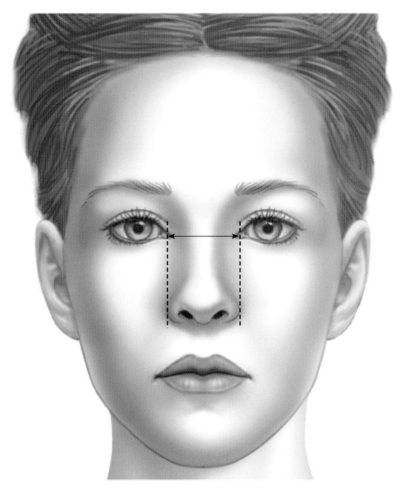

Figure 6-7. Alar width as it approximates the distance between the medial canthi.

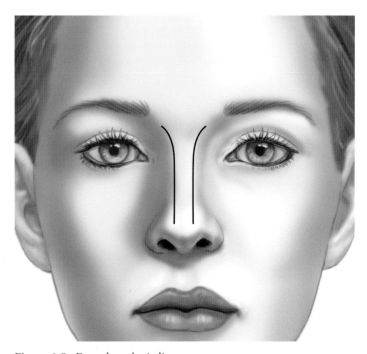

Figure 6-8. Dorsal aesthetic lines.

columella-labial angle or junction, and alar-facial groove or junction (Figure 6-9).

○ *Radix (nasion)*: This point is defined as the junction of the frontal bone and the dorsum of the nose. Two measurements are used to describe the radix: anterior projection and level. The nasion should ideally project approximately 15 mm anterior from the level of the medial canthus and 11 mm anterior to the corneal surface or at a distance 4 mm to 6 mm behind a vertical line tangential through the glabella. The ideal level of the radix should approximate the tarsal edge or the upper lid crease.[9,10]

○ *Dorsum*: On the lateral view, analysis of the nasal dorsum begins at the nasion. Inferior to the nasion, the paired nasal bones may take various forms, either naturally or as the result of trauma. The congenital dorsal hump is often comprised of bone in the superior half and cartilage in the inferior half. The bones themselves may be high or low off the face, shallow or broad, concave or convex, straight or deviated. Their junction medially forms the dorsum. *Low radix disproportion* is a term that refers to a dorsal line that, when seen from the lateral view, begins below the level of the upper eyelid margin when the patient's eyes are held in primary gaze.[11] It is one important cause of nasal imbalance in which the upper part of the nose appears too small in relation to the lower part. The junction between bone and cartilage may be appreciated by identifying the edge of the bones laterally and palpating their course as they extend medially.

○ *Nasofrontal angle*: This angle is formed by intersecting lines between the nasal dorsum and a line parallel to the infrabrow glabella (Figure 6-10). In female patients, the ideal angle is roughly 134 degrees while in male patients the angle is slightly less, about 130 degrees.[12,10] In both genders, the measurement can vary by ethnicity as well.

○ *Nasal tip projection*: Careful analysis of tip projection is important because the final tip projection will dictate the height of the dorsum (Figure 6-11). For this reason, tip projection is achieved before dorsal modification. The appearance of the tip should be evaluated in isolation and as it relates to the nasal dorsum and upper lip. Several methods can be used to measure tip projection and utilizing all three may aid in differentiating the underlying etiology of the problem. Measured from the alar crease to the nasal tip, tip projection should be about two thirds of the distance of nasal length (Figure 6-12). A second measurement is to see if the amount of tip projection approximates the width of the alar base. Finally, if upper lip projection is normal (see nasal orthognathic relationship), a vertical line is drawn tangential to the upper lip, and normal nasal projection is present when between 50% and 60% of the nose is anterior to this line (Figure 6-11).[13,14,15]

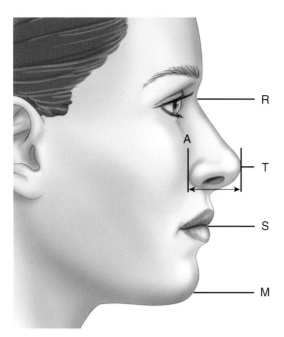

Figure 6-9. Important landmarks on lateral facial profile (R, radix; A, alar groove; T, tip; S, stomion; M, menton).

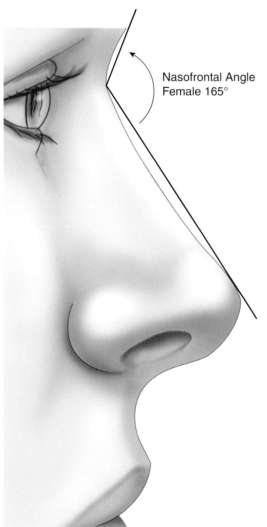

Nasofrontal Angle
Female 165°

Figure 6-10. Normal nasofrontal angle in the female patient.

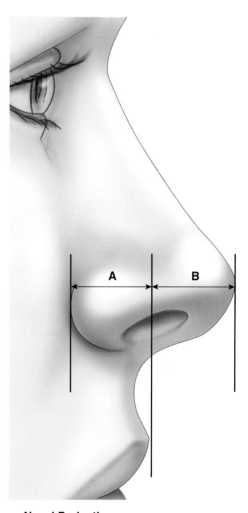

Nasal Projection
A=50-60% of A+B

Figure 6-11. Estimation of normal nasal tip projection.

○ *Nasal length*: The ideal nasal length measured from radix to the tip-defining points should approximate the distance from stomion to menton[16] (Figure 6-9). Another approximation for normal nasal length is that the nasal length to tip projection ratio should be about 1:0.6 (assuming tip projection is normal). The perceived nasal length can be affected by the nasofrontal angle. If the nasofrontal angle is more anterior and superior, the nose may appear longer. In contrast, if the nasofrontal angle is positioned posterior and inferior, the nose may look shorter. The radix may be altered to treat this problem.

○ *Nasolabial angle (tip rotation)*: The caudal extent of the septum and the anterior nasal spine of the midline maxilla are most important in determining the angle between the nasal base and upper lip (Figure 6-13). This relationship is created by the intersection of one tangent along the course of the columella and a second tangent along the upper lip. This angle measures approximately 100 to 105 degrees in females and 90 to 95 degrees in males.[17] Influencing factors on this angle include the upper maxilla, the soft tissue volume of the upper lip, and the inclination of the central dentition. The appearance of the nasolabial angle should be evaluated in repose and with smiling. An acute nasolabial angle and a tip that does not recoil to its prior position after gentle downward pressure indicates a loss of tip support.

○ *Alar-columella relationship*: The lateral view is also a favorable way to evaluate the relationship between the alar rim and the columella (Figure 6-14). Both structures should be curved slightly away from the other, leaving an oval with roughly 2 mm to 3 mm of show on lateral inspection. If one were to bisect the opening axially, an equal amount of columella should be seen above and below this line. Causes of excess columella show include an alar rim that rides too high, a columella that hangs too low, or a combination of the two. Proper treatment begins with identifying the etiology and specifically addressing the cause. Conversely, patients who have too little columellar show might be manifesting a low alar rim, a retracted columella, or a combination of the two.

○ *Chin-lip relationship*: The lower lip and the nose play an important role in chin aesthetics. Several tools can be used to assess chin projection. If nasal length is ideal, a line can be dropped from the mid-dorsum of the nose inferior and tangential to the upper lip. The chin should be about 3 mm posterior to this line according to Byrd.[18] Another method is to drop a line inferior and perpendicular to Frankfurt horizontal that is tangential to the lower lip. The chin should be just posterior to this line in females and at or slightly anterior to it in males. A final analysis is Riedel's line. This line connects the most prominent points of the upper and lower lips. The most prominent point of the chin should be the third point on this line.[19]

○ *Nasal orthognathic relationship*: When a patient presents with concerns about the size of the nose, it is important to assess the position of the jaws and the occlusion of the teeth. It is not uncommon for a patient with complaints about a large nose to in fact have a small mandible or posterior chin point. The retraction of the upper incisors that results from dental compensation allows the upper lip to fall posteriorly, giving the illusion of an overprojected nose. Advancing the mandible or chin as indicated frequently reduces this overprojected appearance.

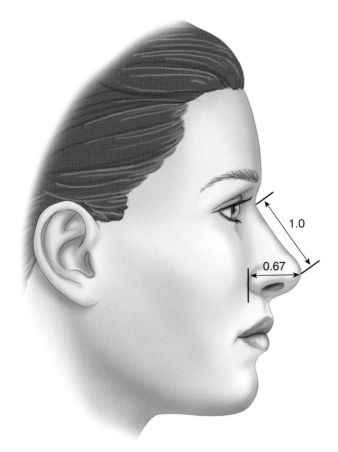

Figure 6-12. Evaluation of nasal length.

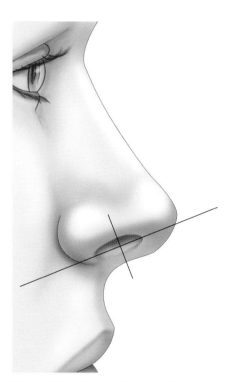

Figure 6-14. Appropriate lateral columellar show.

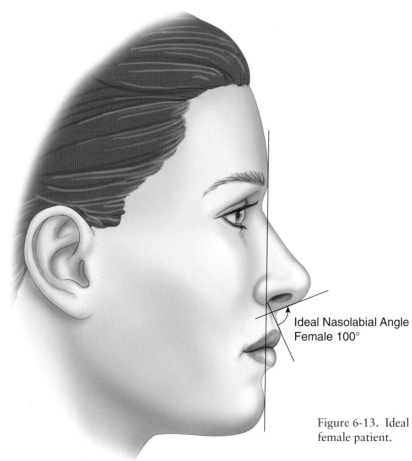

Ideal Nasolabial Angle
Female 100°

Figure 6-13. Ideal nasolabial angle in the female patient.

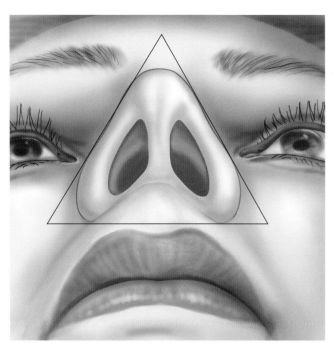

Figure 6-15

- **Worm's eye view:** On basal view, the landmarks should include the infratip lobule, columella, alar sidewall, facet or soft-tissue triangle, nostril sill, nasolabial angle or junction, alar-facial groove or junction, and the tip-defining points.
  - *Alar base:* Inspection of the nose from a "worm's eye" view with the neck extended and the patient gazing skyward is the best way to appreciate the nasal base (Figure 6-15). The nasal base consists of paired and unpaired structures. The columella exists centrally and contains the medial crura of the lower lateral cartilages. The nasal base should approximate an equilateral triangle, and the nostril should be about 50 to 60 degrees relative to a vertical line through the columella. It is bordered by the soft triangles anteriorly, the lateral walls, the alar bases, and the nostril sills. The soft triangles lie anterior to the middle crura and are composed of external skin opposed to internal mucosa. They contain no cartilaginous elements. The nostril sill extends from the terminal extent of the alar rim at the junction of the face to the columella. It may be flat or rolled. The shape of the nostrils is highly variable and usually asymmetric. Their orientation is largely oblique but may be more horizontal or vertical. The ideal nostril-infratip ratio should be between 60:40 to 55:45.[20] The widest point between the alar rims is usually several millimeters superior and lateral to the lateral extent of the nasal sill crease. The width of the alar base should be narrower than the distance between the medial canthi. The boxy nasal tip is characterized by a broad, rectangular appearance of the tip lobule complex.

- Not all ethnicities share the same normative appearances. Variation in nasal anatomy should be recognized and understood.
  - *The African nose:* The African nose is characterized by a dorsum that is wide and shallow with a low radix. Nasal length is shorter and interalar width is greater. The tip exhibits less projection, and because of thicker skin, the tip typically lacks definition. The columellar-labial angle is acute.[21]
  - *The Asian nose:* The Asian nose can be characterized by a low nasal bridge and an underprojected dorsum. Japanese patients may be unique among Asians as having a convex dorsum. Tip projection is less than that of Caucasian noses, and the tip is characterized by a rounded, ill-defined tip that frequently lacks a supratip break. The nasolabial angle is more acute and the alar base tends to be wider than the Caucasian norms. Alar flaring may also be more prominent in Koreans due to variations in the dilator naris muscle.[22]
  - *The Latin nose:* The typical Latin nose was described by Ortiz-Monasterio as having thick skin, a narrow osseocartilaginous vault, minimal tip support, a short columella, and a broad alar base.[23] However, the term "Latin" broadly covers a group of significant ethnic diversity. In the United States with the cultural melange that is unique to our country, the typical Latin nose is not necessarily associated with every Latin patient. Daniel described his observations of Latin diversity in a California practice and found that the Latin nose is on a continuum between the Caucasian nose and that of the Mestizo or Caribbean nose. Therefore, the treatment should be individualized to the patient and their desires.[24]
  - *The Middle Eastern nose:* Rhinoplasty is a popular operation among patients of Middle Eastern descent, and it is important to understand the nuances of the Middle Eastern nose. The dorsum tends to be wide with a dorsal hump, and the radix is typically high and shallow. The tip tends to lack definition and projection. A droopy tip is common among these patients as well. Thick sebaceous skin overlies this anatomy making the Middle Eastern rhinoplasty a challenging endeavor.[25]
- *Similarly, male and female noses have normative differences.*
  - The nasion in females should be lower and more shallow than males.
  - The dorsum in females should be straight or slightly lower than a line drawn from nasal tip to radix.
  - A supratip break is desired on the female nose but may feminize the male nose if overdone.
  - Females can tolerate a narrower nasal base and interalar distance.[17]
- All patients should have preoperative photographs taken. Two-dimensional images provide an excellent

way to logically think about the aesthetics of the face and frequently identify concerns not immediately identified in the examination. Six standard views should be obtained for all patients. These include a square frontal view, two opposing oblique views, two opposing lateral views, and a worm's eye view, which is taken from below placing the tip of the nose between the eyebrows for standard comparison (Figures 6-1 to 6-6). It is important to utilize standardized lighting, object-film distance, and camera settings.[26] With advanced digital SLR cameras, postoperative adjustments can be made to create a 1:1 ratio and compensate for some variation using digital darkroom software such as Adobe Lightroom™ (Adobe Systems Incorporated, San Jose, CA).

- Digital imaging and computer morphing may be helpful aids in helping a patient understand their concerns and goals. Not infrequently a two-dimensional image may allow the surgeon to identify aesthetic abnormalities that were less obvious on the actual physical exam. The patient should be informed that a morphed computer prediction image is not a guarantee of the result but an image to ensure that the patient and surgeon both have the same goals in mind. One should not proceed with the surgery unless the surgeon feels confident that the patient's goals are clearly understood and realistically achievable. If after these techniques, the patient cannot clearly state what he would like to change, it is advisable to decline treating the patient. The surgeon will never be successful correcting something that the patient cannot identify. Historically, there was a fear that a digital image would lead to higher malpractice claims because the patient did not receive the "guaranteed" result; however, these fears have been unsubstantiated.[27] In fact, some experienced surgeons feel that conservative digital morphing may actually lower patient expectations and result in increased satisfaction with the actual result.[28]

- Following direct and photographic examination, the first step is to develop a prioritized problem list. The second step is to tape a piece of clear acetate tracing paper (ordered through any dental supply company or art store) over the patient's photographs and trace in pencil the ideal or desired nasal dimensions. Finally, based on the surgical goals and surgeon's abilities develop an operative plan. It can be useful to mentally perform the surgery and record the steps sequentially on a separate sheet of paper that can be brought to the operating room and placed near the photographs. This surgical plan can then be checked intraoperatively to make sure a step is not missed during the operation. Presurgical operative sequencing also increases the efficiency of the operation by allowing all involved in the operative care to know what the steps are and to have the appropriate materials avail-

able in a timely manner. For more novice surgeons, a conservative management plan should be chosen. Unachievable, unrealistic, or undesirable procedures should be eliminated.

- Rhinoplasty for male patients is common, as men similarly desire improvement in either the appearance or function of the nose. While women are more open about plastic surgery, men tend to be more private. Similar to their female counterparts, male patients may present with displeasure about the appearance of their nose. They may want to alter the size or shape of one or more key components. Men will also present with respiratory issues, such as snoring, related to their nose. While the techniques are similar, the goals for rhinoplasty in the male are different. The acronym "SIMON" (single, immature, male, overly expectant, narcissistic) has been used to denote warning signs of the difficult male patient.[17] If these signs are present, a psychiatric consultation should be considered.

- The surgeon should always be aware of patients with body dysmorphic disorder (BDD). Before considering operative correction, the surgeon should be able to identify the problem of which the patient is concerned and feel capable to address this safely. Patients who are overly concerned with a problem, which the surgeon cannot recognize, may have elements of BDD. These patients will frequently not be satisfied with the results following surgery or turn to another concern, which may or may not be based in fact.

REFERENCES

1. Chait L, Widgerow AD. In search of the ideal nose. *Plast and Reconstr Surg.* 2000;105(7):2561–2567.
2. Farkas L. *Anthropometry of the Head and Face in Medicine.* New York: Elsevier;1981.
3. Patterson CN, Powell DG. Facial analysis in patient evaluation for physiologic and cosmetic surgery. *Laryngoscope* 1974;84:1004.
4. Burres S. Tip points: defining the tip. *Aesthetic Plast Surg.* 1999 Mar–Apr;23(2):113–118.
5. Sheen JH, Sheen AP. *Aesthetic Rhinoplasty.* St. Louis: Mosby; 1978:432–462.
6. Sheen JH and Sheen AP. *Aesthetic Rhinoplasty.* 2nd ed. St. Louis: Mosby; 1987:988–1011.
7. Rohrich RJ, Adams WP Jr. The boxy nasal tip: Classification and management based on alar cartilage suturing techniques. *Plast Reconstr Surg.* 2001 Jun;107(7):1849–1863.
8. Wright WK. Symposium: The supra-tip in rhinoplasty: A dilemma. II. Influence of surrounding structure and prevention. *Laryngoscope* 1976;86:50.
9. Daniel RK. A clinical definition of an ideal radix—Discussion. *Plast Reconstr Surg.* 2002 April:1419.
10. Rohrich R, Muzaffar AR, Janis J. Component dorsal hump reduction: The importance of maintaining dorsal aesthetic lines in rhinoplasty. *Plast Reconstr Surg.* 2004;114:1298.

11. Sheen JH, Sheen AP. *Aesthetic Rhinoplasty*. 2nd ed. St. Louis: Mosby; 1987:808–825.

12. Daniel RK. The radix and the nasofrontal angle. In: Gunter JP, Rohrich RJ, eds. *16th Annual Dallas Rhinoplasty Symposium*. Dallas, TX: University of Texas Southwestern Medical Center; 1999:263.

13. Petroff MA, McCollough EG, Hom D, Anderson JR. Nasal tip projection: Quantitative changes following rhinoplasty. *Arch. Otolaryngol Head Neck Surg.* 1991;117:783.

14. Ricketts, RM. Divine proportion in facial esthetics. *Clin Plast Surg.* 1982;9:401.

15. Gunter JP, Hackney FL. Clinical assessment of facial analysis. In: Gunter JP, Rohrich RJ, Adams WP, eds. *Dallas Rhinoplasty: Nasal Surgery by the Masters*. St. Louis, MO: Quality Medical Publishing; 2002:53–71.

16. Byrd HS, Hobar PC. Rhinoplasty: A practical guide for surgical planning. *Plast Reconstr Surg.* 1993;91:642.

17. Rohrich R, Janis J, Kenkel J. Male rhinoplasty. *Plast Reconstr Surg.* 2003;112:1071.

18. Byrd HS, Burt J. Dimensional approach to rhinoplasty: Perfecting the aesthetic balance between the nose and chin. In: Gunter JP, Rohrich RJ, Adams WP, eds. *Dallas Rhinoplasty: Nasal Surgery by the Masters*. 1st ed. St. Louis, MO: Quality Medical Publishing; 2002.

19. Riedel RA. An analysis of dentofacial relationships. *Am J Orthod.* 1957;43:103.

20. Guyuron B, Ghavami A, Wishnek SM, et al. Components of the short nostril. *Plast Reconstr Surg.* 2005;116:1517.

21. Rohrich R, Muzaffar A. Rhinoplasty in the African American patient. *Plast Reconstr Surg.* 2003;111:1322.

22. Bergeron L, Kuo-Ting. Asian rhinoplasty techniques. In: *Seminars in Plastic Surgery*. New York, NY: Thieme Medical Publishers; 2009:23(1):16.

23. Ortiz-Monasterio F, Olmedo A. Rhinoplasty in the mestizo nose: Secondary rhinoplasty in the thick skinned nose. In Rees TD, Baker DC, Tabbal N (Eds.). *Rhinoplasty: Problems and Controversies*. St Louis, MO: Mosby-Year Book, 1988:372–383.

24. Daniel RK. Hispanic rhinoplasty in the United States, with emphasis on the Mexican American nose. *Plast Reconstr Surg.* 2003;112:244.

25. Rohrich R, Ghavami A. Rhinoplasty for Middle Eastern noses. *Plast Reconstr Surg.* 2009;123:1343.

26. Galdini GM, DaSilva D, Gunter JP. Digital photography for Rhinoplasty. *Plast Reconstr Surg.* 2002;109(4):1421.

27. Muhlbauer W, Holm C. Computer imaging and surgical reality in aesthetic rhinoplasty. *Plast Reconstr Surg.* 2005;115:2098.

28. Gruber R. Realistic expectations: To morph or not to morph—Discussion. *Plast Reconstr Surg.* 2006;119:1352.

Chapter 7. Treatment Planning: Nasal Function

- *Nasal function*: For numerous reasons, breathing through the nose is more beneficial than breathing through the mouth. Humidification occurs as the air passes from the nose to the lungs. In fact, 90% of humidification occurs before the air reaches the lungs across the turbinates (Figures 7-1 and 7-2). Air can be heated as much as 25°C to 30°C during inspiration, and the nose plays a large role in thermal regulation.[1,2] Particulate filtration occurs in the nasal vibrissae just inside the nares where large particles may be trapped. Impingement is a process where smaller particles are filtered, and the two areas where this occurs are the internal nasal valve and the posterior nasopharynx. The mucociliary system also plays a major role in particulate filtration.[3]

- *Nasal physiology*: As one breathes through the nose, the regular pace of the respiratory cycle is maintained. Afferent stimuli from nerve endings in the nose travel to the brain to control the rhythm and rate of breathing. Additionally, the brain senses the efflux of carbon dioxide and responds by maintaining a normal tone in the pulmonary vasculature and a normal production of mucus. Breathing through the mouth bypasses these nerve endings, disrupting the respiratory cycle and stimulating the brain to produce larger amounts of mucus and increase pulmonary vascular resistance. Chronic increases in vascular resistance lead to pulmonary hypertension. With expiration, air exits the nose across a smaller cross-sectional area, which creates back-pressure in the respiratory tree. This keeps the terminal alveoli open longer permitting more time for gas exchange. Too rapid a loss of carbon dioxide, as occurs with hyperventilation, alters the pH of the blood.[4]

- *Nasal cycle*: Normally, there is a cyclical enlargement and contraction of the nasal mucosa that alternates between nostrils: When one side is engorging, the other is contracting. This cycle may take between 1 and 5 hours and its purpose is unknown.[3]

- *History*: Many factors are considered in elucidating the etiology of nasal obstructive symptoms: duration, frequency, laterality, and seasonality. The patient should be questioned about a history of trauma, allergies, and medications. Seasonal or geographic symptoms are typical of a disorder that is best treated medically. Obstruction only in deep inspiration or heavy breathing is characteristic of a collapsed internal nasal valve, whereas an obstruction that is constant is indicative of a fixed mechanical obstruction such as an enlarged turbinate or septal deviation.

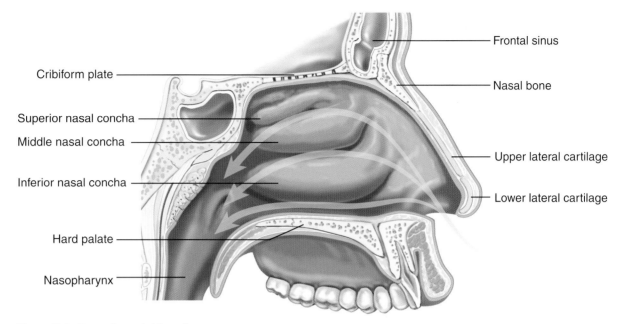

Figure 7-1. Lateral nasal sidewall anatomy.

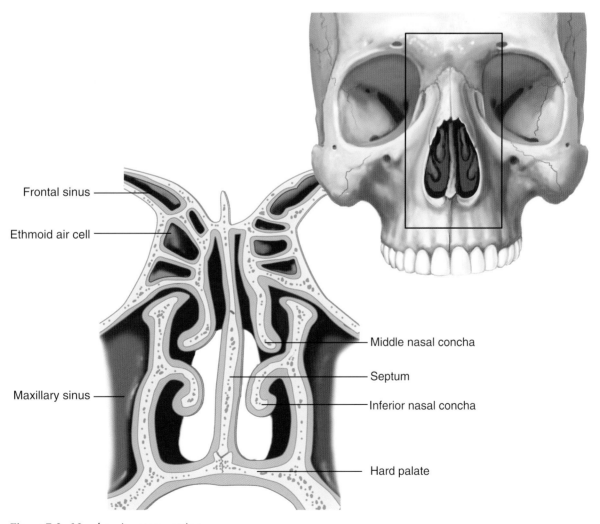

Figure 7-2. Nasal cavity cross-section.

- *External examination*: Examination of the nasal morphology may reveal potential sources of airflow obstruction.
  - The lower lateral cartilages provide support to the alar rims and serve to keep the external nasal valves open (Figure 7-3). Any abnormalities or collapse of this external nasal valve with inspiration should be noted and evaluated. The static position of the septum from a worm's eye view should be noted. Caudal deviation may be noted by visualization of the caudal edge of the septum within either of the two nostrils. Nasal deviation from frontal view may also be indicative of an obstructive septal deviation.
  - The skin over the internal nasal valve should also be noted with and without deep inspiration. Medial excursion of this skin may be indicative of internal valve collapse. Simple observation should note whether these valves remain open or collapse on inspiration, indicating the degree to which the lower lateral cartilages provide adequate alar support.
  - The Cottle maneuver is an additional test to identify compromise of the internal nasal valve (Figure 7-4). The patient is asked to breathe in and out through the nose while the opposite nostril is held closed. This breathing is done with and without lateral traction on the cheek. Any difference in the ease of respiration is noted, and "significant" improvement in respiration is taken as a positive test. Gruber et al. reported improved accuracy in diagnosing nasal valve compromise using commercially available strips to individually spread the upper and lower lateral cartilages to separately evaluate internal and external valves, respectively.[5]

Outer nasal vault

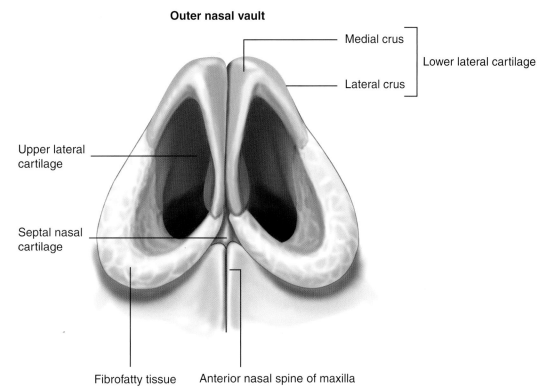

Medial crus

Lateral crus

Lower lateral cartilage

Upper lateral cartilage

Septal nasal cartilage

Fibrofatty tissue

Anterior nasal spine of maxilla

Figure 7-3. Nasal base on worm's eye view.

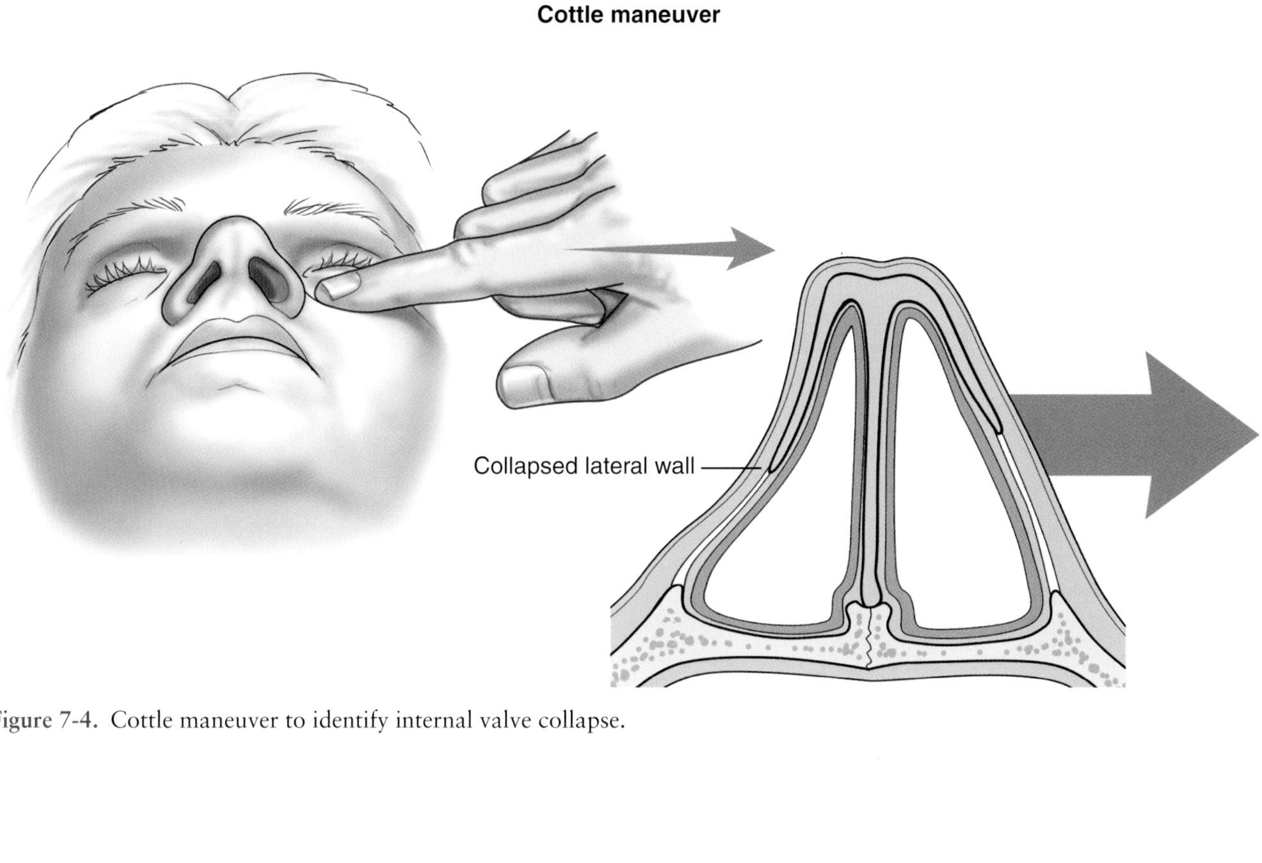

Cottle maneuver

Collapsed lateral wall

Figure 7-4. Cottle maneuver to identify internal valve collapse.

- *Intranasal examination*: Using a nasal speculum and adequate lighting, the internal anatomy of the nose should always be assessed. This should be performed before and after use of a vasoconstrictive agent, such as oxymetazoline. Any scar tissue, webs, or narrowing should be identified. These may affect blood flow through either the external or internal nasal valve. The angle the upper lateral cartilages make with the septum should also be noted (Figures 7-5). An angle of 15 degrees or greater is felt to be adequate for unimpeded airflow. Examination while the patient inspires may provide additional evidence of compromised function.
  - The position of the more central septum should be noted, taking care to describe any defects or deformity. Deformities of the septum may be in the anterior-posterior plane, the sagittal plane, or a combination of both. The caudal border may rest in the center of the anterior nasal spine or lateral to it. The caudal margin may be palpated through the overlying columellar skin and soft tissue. A cotton-tipped applicator is used to palpate the septum and determine if sufficient stock exists for graft harvest. The presence, size, and location of any septal perforations should be documented as well.
  - The turbinates comprise the bulk of the surface area of the nasal mucosa and play an integral role in respiration. There are three stacked turbinates in the superior-inferior plane. The inferior turbinate is the most visible when looking into the vestibule and is the most responsible for altering nasal airflow. The middle and superior turbinates are more difficult to visualize.
- Swelling of the nasal turbinates, due to allergy or exposure to environmental irritants, may lead to blockage of the airway. Treatment of the underlying cause may reduce the swelling but often more drastic measures are indicated. Generally, because the turbinates are essential for respiration, only small amounts of turbinate tissue should be removed.

- Some surgeons routinely measure nasal airflow and pressure during respiration preoperatively and postoperatively by rhinomanometry. This serves to quantify the amount of existing resistance and the improvement following surgery. Symptomatic patients generally record values above 0.3 Pa/mL/s.[6] Active rhinomanometry measures flow and resistance from the normal respiratory cycle.[7] It samples data from either a sensor just inside the nasal vestibule, in the nasopharynx, or in the oropharynx. Acoustic rhinometry is a newer type of rhinometry that measures airflow based on acoustic reflections noninvasively.[8] In general, nasal obstruction may result from either hypertrophy of the mucosa, altered nasal anatomy, or a combination of the two. A mucosal etiology is suggested by diminution in resistance following use of a nasal decongestant.

REFERENCES

1. Ballenger JJ. Symposium: The nose versus the environment. *Laryngoscope*. 1983;93:56.
2. Weiner JS. Nose shape and climate. *Am J Phys Anthropol*. 1954;12(4):615–618.
3. Howard B, Rohrich R. Understanding the nasal airway: Principles and practice. *Plast Reconstr Surg*. 2002; 109:1128.
4. Cottle MH. Nasal breathing pressures and cardio-pulmonary illness. *Eye Ear Nose Throat Mon*. 1972;51(9): 331–340.
5. Gruber RP, Lin AY, Richards T. A predictive test and classification for valvular nasal obstruction using nasal strips. *Plast Reconstr Surg*. 2010 Jul;126(1):143–145.
6. Bailey B, ed. Nasal function and evaluation, nasal obstruction. In: *Head and Neck Surgery: Otolaryngology*. 2nd ed. New York, NY: Lippincott-Raven; 1998:335–344,376, 380–390.
7. Kerr A, ed. Rhinology. In: *Scott-Brown's Otolaryngology*. 6th ed. Oxford: Butterworth-Heinemann; 1997. Active
8. Grymer LF. Reduction rhinoplasty and nasal patency: Change in the cross sectional area of the nose evaluated by acoustic rhinometry. *Laryngoscope*. 1995;105:429.

Inner nasal vault

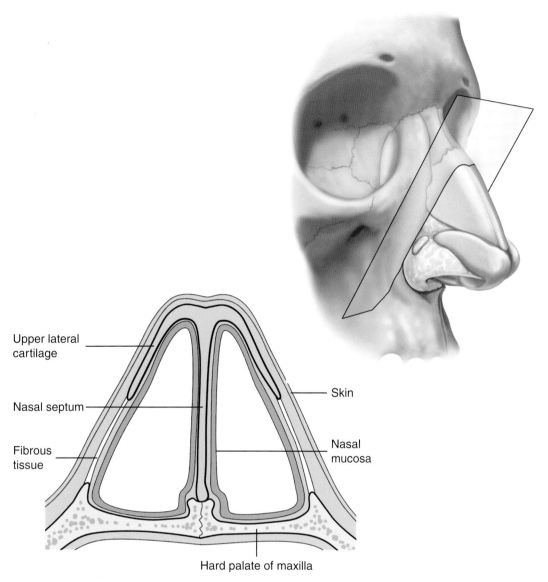

Upper lateral cartilage

Skin

Nasal septum

Nasal mucosa

Fibrous tissue

Hard palate of maxilla

Figure 7-5. Nasal cavity at the level of the internal nasal valve shown above.

Chapter 8. Operative Setup

- Rhinoplasty is best performed in a supine or head-up position on an operating room bed or flexed operating chair. A circular cushion is placed at the occiput to support the head and a shoulder roll is placed transversely behind the shoulders to gently extend the neck. The arms are placed at the sides with padding beneath the elbows to avoid ulnar nerve injury due to prolonged compression.

- Lighting is of key importance since certain structures may be hidden in shadow beneath overlying soft tissue. Overhead operating lights are often insufficient and a headlight is recommended. This allows the surgeon to direct a focused beam of light onto the working area. Suction/irrigation devices with a light incorporated into the tip may also be useful.

- Anesthesia for rhinoplasty is largely determined by surgeon preference and the need for adjunctive procedures. Local anesthesia with or without intravenous sedation may be perfectly adequate for many patients and may be administered safely. This is typically indicated for modification of the soft tissues rather than osteotomies. Intravenous propofol may be used and titrated to a level of adequate sedation without losing spontaneous respiration. Many patients and surgeons alike prefer general anesthesia because it minimizes patient sensation during the procedure and allows the anesthesiologist to safely control the patient's blood pressure as a means of minimizing blood loss. If bleeding is to be expected, a protected airway is advantageous in that it reduces the chance of laryngospasm. The sedated patient is breathing spontaneously, and the protective cough reflex is blunted. If blood or irrigation lands on the vocal cords, laryngospasm may be induced, creating an airway emergency. With a secure airway, this potential complication can be avoided. The need to harvest bone or cartilage from a remote site, such as calvarium or rib, also makes general anesthesia a preferable choice. If general anesthesia is chosen, the endotracheal tube (ETT) or laryngeal mask airway (LMA) is best taped so that it does not interfere with exposure of the tip or osteotomies. An ETT or LMA that is taped at the corner of the mouth may pull the oral commissure and thus the nasal tip resulting in a tip deviation that may confound the surgeon's ability to assess tip symmetry.

- In addition to setting up the operative instruments on a larger sterile table, a small prep table should be used. This should include a speculum, small scissors, Bacitracin, as well as an antimicrobial solution, pledgets soaked in a vasoconstrictive solution, a 10 cc syringe with 1% lidocaine with 1/100,000 epinephrine, and a 1½ inch 25-gauge needle. The speculum is used to confirm the preoperative findings from the intranasal examination.

- The nasal hairs are trimmed with scissors (or a #15 scalpel blade) to improve visualization and avoid entrapment of hair within the incisions. The vestibules are then prepped with an antimicrobial solution such as a dilute iodine solution. Lidocaine with epinephrine is then injected into the columella, lateral nasal walls, dorsum, tip, intranasally, and into the septum if a septoplasty is to be performed. It is important to inject prior to the surgical prep and drape so the epinephrine has completely taken effect prior to incision. The authors typically inject about 8 cc to 10 cc. Immediately after injection, the nose will appear amorphous, but by the time the prep and draping is complete the fluid has been absorbed and redistributed returning the nose to its normal anatomy. The nares are then packed with cotton pledgets soaked in a vasoconstrictive agent as indicated. A 4% cocaine solution may be safely used in most instances. The pledgets are left in place for 7 to 10 minutes and removed at the start of the procedure. It may be helpful to trim the strings attached to the pledgets so that they are not inadvertently removed during prepping. If cocaine solution is not available or desired, oxymetazoline may be used as a substitute. Additional injection of an anesthetic/vasoconstrictive solution is also recommended if the septum requires manipulation. Hydrodissection of the septal mucosa off the cartilage is done with the syringe and 25-gauge needle immediately before dissection.

- Around the pledgets, the face is prepped with any of the standard solutions, such as dilute iodine-povidone solution or chlorhexidine. Care should be taken to avoid exposure keratitis with an ophthalmologic safe lubrication before prepping and avoiding pooling of fluid around the eyes. If the oral cavity is not to be entered, it may be sealed off from the operative site with a sterile transparent dressing. Generally, scleral shields are not required for rhinoplasty. A small Tegaderm cut in half will seal the eyes shut, while leaving access to the medial nose for clinical assessment and osteotomy access. If cranial bone graft is planned, the entire head needs to be prepped and the area over the proposed incision infiltrated. If costal bone/cartilage grafts are required, a separate area over the chest needs to be prepped and infiltrated.

- Unlike other procedures, the bulk of instruments used for rhinoplasty are highly specialized and developed for specific operative maneuvers.
  - *Nasal speculum*: various sizes should be available to examine the nose under anesthesia at the start of the procedure and provide retraction of soft tissue during the procedure.
  - #11 and #15 scalpel blades.
  - *Iris scissors*: useful for dissection of the lower lateral cartilages and excision of the cephalic portion for volume reduction and tip definition.
  - *Fine double-hook retractor*: useful to separate the medial crura of the lower lateral cartilages to approach the caudal septum.
  - *Large double-ball and double-hook retractor*: useful when placed on the nasal rim for exposure of the distal nasal mucosa to identify the course of the intranasal incision.
  - *Cottle elevator*: long, narrow instrument with a small circular paddle with sharp edges at one end. It is used to dissect mucosa or perichondrium or periosteum off cartilage or bone. The shaft is marked in one-centimeter increments so that it can be used to measure certain depths.
  - *Aufricht retractor*: angled retractor of adequate width to expose the bony and cartilaginous nasal dorsum. When exposing the dorsum, it should be noted that adjacent structures are pulled out of place.
  - *Goldman elevator*: thick, straight elevator with blunt edges used to out-fracture the nasal bones.
  - *Freer elevator*: small, fine paddle used to elevate periosteum off underlying bone.
  - *Brown-Adson forceps*: small-toothed forceps useful for handling cartilage since multiple, small teeth minimize large perforations.
  - *Ballinger blade (swivel knife)*: used to excise central portions of septal cartilage once the mucosa has been elevated off either side of the septum. The blade is used by contacting the caudal and superior corner of the portion of cartilage to be resected, pushing the handle posteriorly (while preserving one centimeter of dorsal septum), contacting the anterior edge of the ethmoid, changing direction of the swivel blade by pressing inferiorly on the handle, and finally pulling anterior along the vomer to cut the remaining inferior edge of septum and deliver the graft material.
  - *Rasps*: tools with a jagged end that come in a variety of styles. Pull and push rasps act as their names imply. The latter shave bone off a fixed structure such as the bony dorsum when it is pushed across the surface. The former only works in a pulling direction. Mild or moderate reduction is best performed with a rasp to prevent overreduction. More significant reduction may be performed with a controlled osteotomy of the nasal bones. A Rubin chisel may be used to prevent an unequal bony reduction.
  - *Nasal osteotomes*: the classic nasal osteotomes are paired, a right-sided osteotome and a left-sided osteotome. Each is curved to assist in performing a low position to mid or high position osteotomy. Depending on the manufacturer, one side of the groove is sharp while the opposite side is blunt. This is to minimize trauma to the skin as one follows the leading edge superiorly along the maxilla. Generally, nondisplaced injury to the internal mucosa heals without adverse sequelae.
  - Symmetrical guarded osteotome for larger reductions of the bony dorsum.
  - Suture material is largely personal preference. Some prefer absorbable material since the suture disappears over time and is less prone to eventual "spitting." Others prefer nonabsorbable material, such as clear nylon or Prolene, which provide long-term support but may palpable or lead to suture granulomas. For cartilage grafts, 5-0 PDS offers good long-term support but ultimately resorbs reducing the incidence of a suture-related complication. Both 4-0 and 5-0 sutures are appropriate for suturing cartilage. The rim incisions can be closed with 5-0 chromic gut and the columella closed with 5-0 Vicryl and 6-0 nylon for the subcutaneous tissue and skin, respectively.
  - PDS flexible plate (Mentor Worldwide LLC) is a new material that is made from polydioxanone, a resorbable material that is degraded by hydrolysis and absorbed by the body. Polydioxanone has been used for years for bone defects.[1] This material is now available as a flexible plate in various thicknesses: 0.15 mm, 0.25 mm, and 0.5 mm. The thinner sheets are useful to serve as a scaffold to link small pieces of cartilage into a larger piece. The thicker sheets have enough rigidity to straighten warped cartilage, reinforce weak cartilage, or be used as a septal extension graft to aid in tip positioning that can be reinforced with tip sutures and additional grafts.
- *Tips*:
  - The setup for rhinoplasty surgery uses unique instruments and each surgeon will have a personal setup. It is useful to have a laminated photograph of the instrument set up for the nurses to reference in order to make sure all the instruments are available and set up in the desired arrangement. This is true for the main table as well as the back preparation table.

REFERENCE

1. Hollinger JO, Battistone GC. Biodegradable bone repair materials: Synthetic polymers and ceramics. *Clin Orthop Relat Res.* 1986;207:290.

Chapter 9. Basic Approaches

- The right-handed surgeon should stand on the right side of the operating room table to facilitate manipulation through both the right and left nares with either the head in a neutral position or gently moved from side to side.
- *Open Approach*: The open approach to rhinoplasty involves exposure of the subcutaneous structures by incising the skin across the columella, continuing the incision along the mucocutaneous junction behind the columella, upwards behind the soft triangles, and then around just inferior to the caudal edge of the lower lateral cartilages. In the technique described, the entire nasal covering is elevated so that specific maneuvers may be performed to restructure and reshape the nose.
  - The choice of incision across the columella is purely one of preference and is placed roughly at the narrowest portion. Some surgeons prefer a stair-step incision (Figure 9-1), while others prefer a gull-wing–shaped incision (Figure 9-2). A straight line is usually avoided since the scar often remains more noticeable. A #15 scalpel blade is used for the horizontal portions of the incision and can certainly be used for the entire incision, however. The pointed tip of a #11 blade is often preferable for the vertical portion with the incision in this limb made with a controlled stabbing motion. Care must be taken not to damage the underlying medial crura of the lower lateral cartilages. These often lie close to the skin surface and are prone to injury when incising the skin.
  - It is important to create a 90-degree transition from the horizontal portion of the incision across the columella to the vertical portion along the mucocutaneous junction behind it (Figure 9-3). This will help maintain the integrity of the columella by again minimizing contracture as well as visibility of the scar. It is helpful to mark this 90-degree angle to ensure its accuracy.
  - To provide adequate exposure, the mucosal incisions along the medial borders of the columella need to be continued around the alar rims of the nostrils. This is usually at the level of the inferior aspect of the lateral crus of the lower lateral cartilage but may be performed at various levels (Figure 9-4). The position of this incision relates to the underlying lower lateral cartilages. The most common incision is a rim incision that parallels the inferior border of the lateral crus of the lower lateral cartilage. It is important to note that this incision follows the lower lateral cartilage, so it should progress cephalad (away from the nostril edge) as it proceeds laterally. This superolateral direction of the lower lateral cartilage can be seen as a ridge through the vestibular skin. Incisions placed within the substance of the lower lateral cartilage ("intracartilaginous incision") parallel to its main axis or along the superior border of the lower lateral cartilage just behind the inferior border of the upper lateral cartilage ("intercartilaginous incision") are used when a closed technique is chosen.

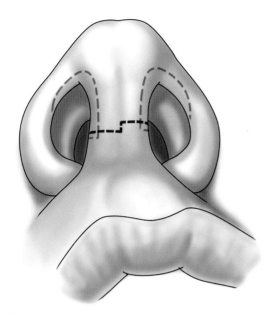

Figure 9-1. Stair-step type incision across the columella.

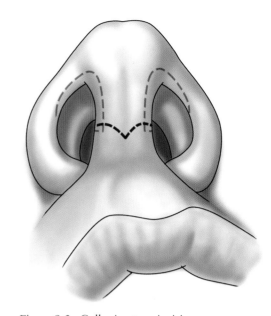

Figure 9-2. Gull-wing type incision.

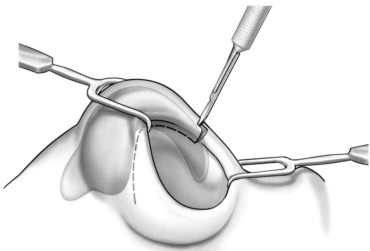

Figure 9-3. Transition of the columella incision from anterior to lateral.

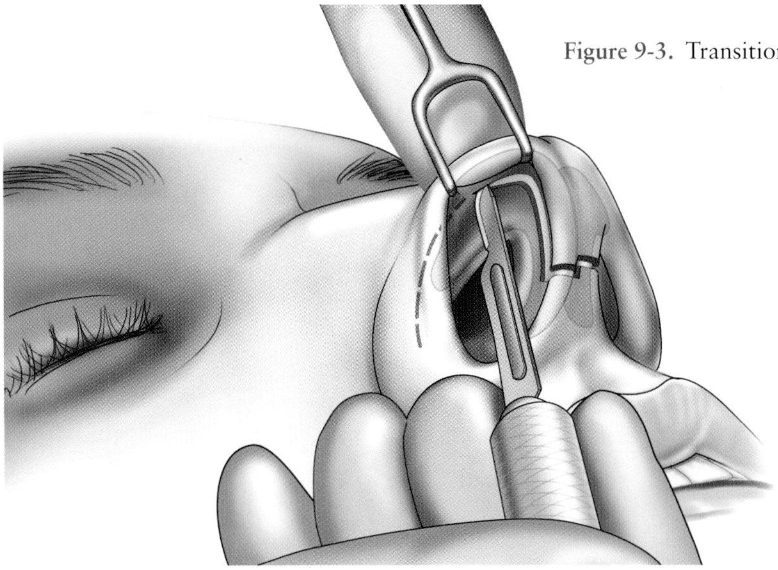

Figure 9-4. Alar rim portion of the incision along the inferior margin of the lower lateral cartilage.

○ Once the incisions are made, a sharp iris scissors is advanced beneath the columellar incision from right to left in a plane between the underlying cartilage and the subcutaneous tissue. Placing a gloved finger over the skin of the columella and palpating the scissor tip as it crosses from one side to the other will determine the correct depth since the scissors will be palpable beneath the skin if they are kept superficial to the cartilage. With gentle spreading of the scissor tips, the correct plane is created. The scissor tips should exit on the left side of the columella within the vertical incision already made with the scalpel (Figure 9-5). The skin is then completely incised with the scissors protecting the cartilage below and retracted superiorly.

○ Care should be taken not to grasp the thin tip of the columella but rather to retract it with a fine double hook as the underlying soft tissues are divided. The plane above the lower lateral cartilages is identified and followed superiorly onto the tip. Placing the tips of the scissors directly onto the surface of the cartilages and gently spreading the soft tissues will determine the correct plane, which is just above the perichondrium (Figure 9-6). Laterally, dissection can be initiated by placing the tips of a curved iris scissors perpendicular to the incision line and gently spreading. One tip should be just inferior to the caudal edge of the lower lateral cartilage and the other against the opposing edge if the incision. This maneuver should easily provide entrance into the proper dissection plane. The white color of the lower lateral cartilages should be easily visible.

The middle and lateral crura are often more substantial than the medial crura, making identification somewhat easier (Figure 9-7). Soft tissue dissection should be directly on the surface of the cartilage and all soft tissue elevated from it. This plane facilitates a dry operative field and minimizes postoperative bruising. The soft tissue between the lower lateral cartilages is excised as dissection proceeds towards the nasal tip.

○ Using a double-prong hook and a finger to evert the skin, excess fibrofatty tissue can be removed from the tip, if necessary. Caution should be taken to not damage the subdermal plexus and gentle cautery used to control bleeding so as not to injure the overlying skin. A needle tip cautery set between 10 to 15 works well.

○ Dissection of the dorsum is frequently performed with scissors, keeping the tips immediately over the dorsal septum caudally and then the nasal bones as the surgeon moves towards the glabella. The soft tissues are elevated off the dorsal supporting structures, and too much lateral dissection should be avoided if osteotomies are to be performed. Some soft tissue attachment should be left on the bones to hold them in place following infracture. A freely dissected nasal bone risks greater malposition after fracture.

○ Once fully freed, an Aufricht retractor may be inserted into the space over the dorsum to provide exposure to the midline structures. A wide double hook may be placed beneath the soft triangles and pulled inferiorly to provide additional exposure.

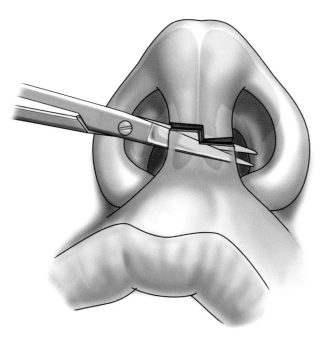

Figure 9-5. Fine iris scissor being passed under the skin and over the lower lateral cartilages.

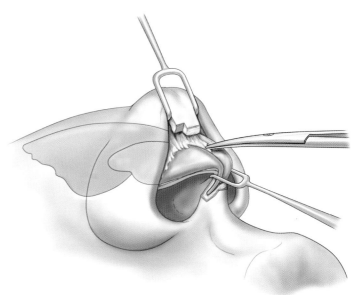

Figure 9-6. Elevation of the soft tissue off the perichondrium of the lower lateral cartilage.

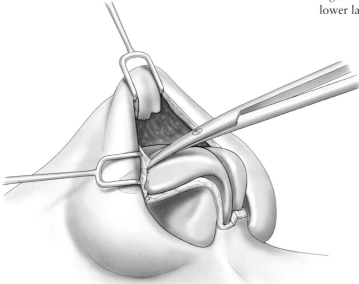

Figure 9-7. Exposure of the nasal tip above the lower lateral cartilages.

- *Closed ("endonasal") Technique*: The endonasal technique must address the same anatomical structures and areas of concern as the open technique. It must be able to expose the dorsum and nasal cartilages. It must also be able to expose and allow manipulation of the septal cartilage, either for reconstruction or harvest.
  - A transfixion incision is made through the nasal mucosa caudal to the nasal septum within the nasal vestibule (Figure 9-8). If no tip work is required, a hemi-transfixion incision may be used, which spares the opposite nasal mucosa and exposes only the septum.
  - The external portions of the nose are degloved with bilateral infra- and intercartilaginous incisions around the lateral crura of the lower lateral cartilages. These are then extended medially above the nasal valve and around the septal angle to meet the superior extent of the transfixion incision(s).
  - Through these incisions, the soft tissue over the dorsum and upper lateral cartilages may be dissected in a subperichondrial plane with a scissors (Figure 9-9). To separate the dorsum into its component parts, a scalpel may be used to divide the mucosa and upper lateral cartilages from the septum. Healing, however, may result in scarring and constriction of the internal nasal valve. Therefore, preservation of the mucosa should be preferred. The dorsal structures once free can be taken down together or separated above the mucosa.
  - To address the nasal tip, the paired infracartilaginous, and intercartilaginous incisions create two bipedicle flaps of nasal mucosa and lower lateral cartilage (Figure 9-10). These may be delivered outside the skin envelope for better visualization and ease of manipulation. Portions of the lower lateral cartilages may be resected and sutures placed—both within each cartilage and between the two cartilages—to change the shape and form of the nasal tip (Figure 9-11).
  - An intracartilaginous incision may also be used to perform a closed reduction of the cephalic portions of the lower lateral cartilages. Using a 25-gauge needle and methylene blue ink, the proposed incision may be marked. The needle is passed through the skin of the alar rim and into the nostril 6 mm to 8 mm above the inferior border of the cartilage being careful to leave enough cartilage behind for rim support. With the needle through the skin, cartilage, and mucosa, it is dipped in ink and withdrawn from the nose. This is repeated along the alar rim until several points have been made along the mucosa. The proposed incision is then seen along the inner nasal mucosa and completed with a scalpel through mucosa and cartilage, stopping short of the skin. Retraction and protection may be afforded by placing a double hook on the edge of the alar rim and pressing the mucosa outwards with a gloved finger. Once through the cartilage along the proposed

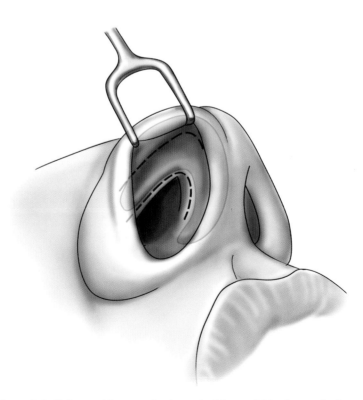

Figure 9-8. Infra- and intercartilaginous incisions within the vestibule.

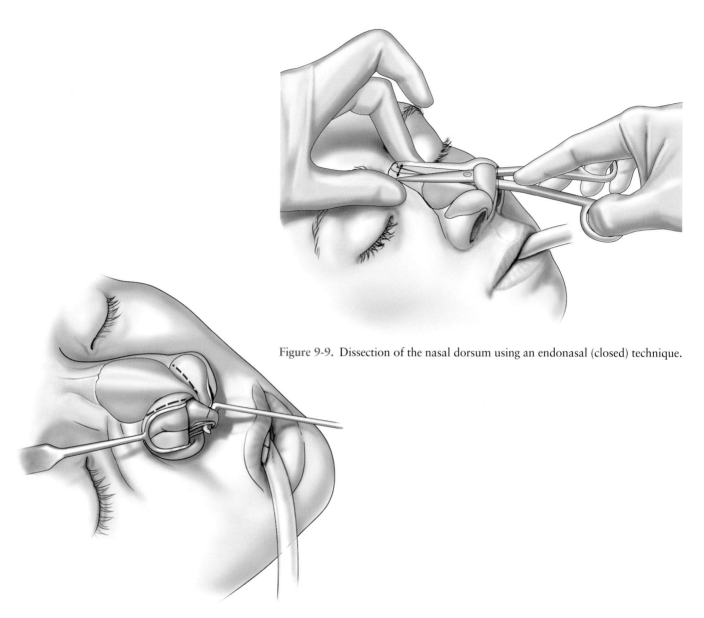

Figure 9-9. Dissection of the nasal dorsum using an endonasal (closed) technique.

Figure 9-10. Delivery of a bipedicle flap of nasal mucosa and cartilage using an endonasal delivery technique.

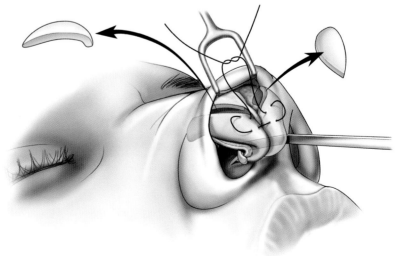

Figure 9-11. Cephalic trim and spanning sutures placed in the lower lateral cartilage using an endonasal delivery technique.

length of the incision, dissection may proceed superiorly above and below the more cephalic portion of cartilage to be resected.

- *Septal Exposure*: If the septum needs to be manipulated or harvested for graft material, it may be approached in one of several ways, depending on whether an open or closed approach is used.
  - *Open rhinoplasty septal harvest*:
    - *Caudal approach*: The caudal septum may be identified by separating the lower lateral cartilages during an open approach (Figure 9-12). After dividing the ligamentous structures between the medial and middle crura, retraction will expose the caudal portion of the septal cartilage. A light touch of the needle tip cautery (set at 10) will expose the cartilage beneath the perichondrium and aid in establishing a dry dissection plane. The septal mucosa is tightly adherent anteriorly and dissection should proceed cautiously (Figures 9-13 and 9-14). This approach also allows the surgeon access to suture the middle and medial cartilages to the caudal septum if repositioning of the tip is necessary. It is important to remember to reestablish tip support upon closing by using medial crural sutures and/or a columellar strut graft.
    - *Dorsal approach*: The septum may also be visualized from above by separating the upper lateral cartilages from their attachments to the septum (Figure 9-15). The dorsal septum is identified anterior to the upper lateral cartilages, and the dorsal edge is brushed with a needle tip cautery to create dry exposure to the cartilage. A subperichondrial dissection is now started with a sharp Cottle elevator just 3 mm to 4 mm below the dorsal edge of the septum. It is useful to use a Brown-Adson forceps to stabilize the flimsy septum while this dissection is initiated. Once this plane has been established, the Cottle is used to dissect in a posterior direction along the superior edge of the dorsal septum. This dissection is blind in that the Cottle is now tunneling directly beneath the upper lateral cartilages. Once these tunnels have been created bilaterally, a #15 blade is placed adjacent to the septum and just inferior to the upper lateral cartilage with the sharp edge facing in a superior direction. The blade is then elevated to separate the medial aspect of the upper lateral cartilage from the dorsal septum all the way to the nasal bones. At this point, the Cottle is used more posteriorly to establish wide subperichondrial undermining from the septum in the posterior two thirds of the septum where this dissection is relatively easy. Once the posterior two thirds of the septal mucosa has been elevated, the dissection proceeds carefully in an anterior direction to complete the dissection. As soon as there is enough room, a speculum can be placed on either side of the septum to spread the dissected mucosa from the septum facilitating exposure to the operative field.
  - Occasionally in an open rhinoplasty, the surgeon may opt to harvest septal cartilage in a manner similar to that described below for closed rhinoplasty. This instance could be a complex tip requiring direct exposure but not access to the entire dorsum.

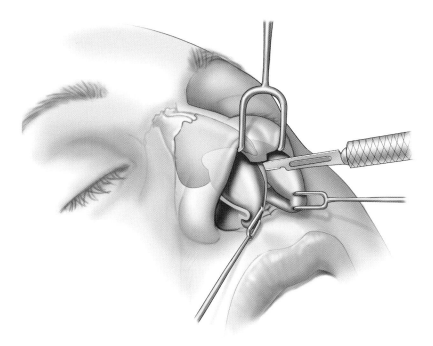

Figure 9-12. Opening the perichondrium over the septum.

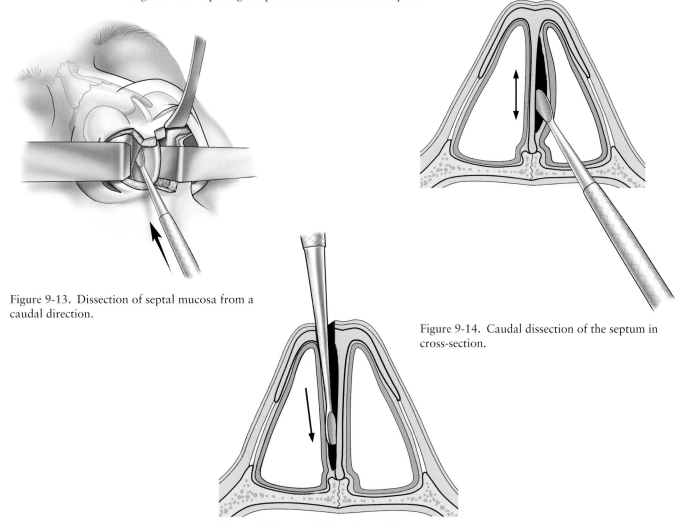

Figure 9-13. Dissection of septal mucosa from a caudal direction.

Figure 9-14. Caudal dissection of the septum in cross-section.

Figure 9-15. Dorsal dissection of the septum in cross-section.

○ *Closed rhinoplasty septal harvest*:

- If approached through the nostril, the mucosal incision is made at or posterior to the caudal edge (Figure 9-16). This is easily identified by deflecting the columella to the left. Once the mucosa is incised, a Freer or Cottle elevator is used to dissect off the mucosa on the right side of the septum. The dissection should proceed posteriorly to the perpendicular plate of the ethmoid, which will have a different feel than cartilage, and inferiorly to the vomer (Figure 9-17). Once the right side is dissected, the sharper end of the Freer or a Cottle elevator may be used to incise the septum in a vertical direction 1 cm off the caudal edge. The nasal mucosa on the contralateral left side should be preserved. The opposite side of the septal cartilage is then dissected in a similar fashion to isolate the septal cartilage. In difficult dissections, it may be impossible to avoid tears in the septal mucosa. As long as these are small and occur only on one side of the mucosa, a septal perforation should not develop. However, if tears occur on each side that are opposite of each other, a septal perforation will occur if the mucosal tears are not repaired. In this case, repairs can be made by suturing the torn mucosa to adjacent intact mucosa. With adequate mobilization of the mucosa, each blade of a nasal speculum may be placed between the septum and mucosa for exposure. Next, a desired graft of cartilage may be harvested. With the anterior incision already completed, the superior incision may be made with a scalpel scissors, or Ballenger blade (swivel knife) parallel to the nasal dorsum, cognizant that at least a 1-cm strut of cartilage be left for support. The posterior and inferior incisions are often better performed with the Ballenger blade. The graft is removed with a cartilage forceps. Once adequate cartilage has been harvested, one or more chromic mattress sutures should be placed across the septum to minimize development of a hematoma in the dead space between the sides of nasal mucosa.

○ It is important to remember that whenever septal cartilage is harvested, at least 1 cm of cartilage needs to remain intact at the caudal and dorsal borders to maintain nasal support. If a fracture of this cartilage occurs during the dissection, it needs to be sutured together to maintain its integrity. The PDS foil is useful to reinforce these repairs when they occur.

○ When a smaller volume of septal cartilage is required, a localized portion can be removed from the septum. In such instances, the entire graft can be visualized and harvested 1 cm below the dorsal edge with a scalpel, in lieu of the Ballinger swivel knife.

○ Posterior to the cartilaginous septum is the perpendicular plate of the ethmoid bone. This may or may not be deviated, but can serve as graft material. It is often strong enough to support warped septal cartilage. Prior to use, it should be perforated with a narrow caliber drill to permit ingrowth and minimize malposition and resorption. The perforations can also be used to hold sutures.

- *Pitfalls*:

  ○ The columellar skin comes quite close the medial footplates of the lower lateral cartilages. Care should be taken when using a scalpel in this area and making sure the scissor tips ride over the cartilage to prevent cartilage injury.

  ○ Non-Caucasian patients are prone to undesirable scarring across the columella. Synechiae and webbing may develop within the nasal vestibule along mucosal incisions. Precise skin closure is paramount.

  ○ Defatting of the soft tissues should not be relied upon to provide better definition of the nasal tip, and damage to the subdermal plexus by aggressive defatting should be avoided. In patients with thicker, more glabrous skin, removal of fat from the tip will often do little to provide better refinement.

- *Tips*:

  ○ Careful attention should be paid to the transition between the horizontal cutaneous portion of the incision and the vertical mucosal portion of the incision within the columella. This should be a true right angle, marked preoperatively and reconstructed meticulously at the conclusion of the procedure.

  ○ A wide double-hook retractor should be used to expose the intranasal portion of the incision.

  ○ The area at the soft triangle is the most difficult to visualize. By using a finger to evert this area with a skin hook, exposure is optimized.

  ○ It may be easiest to dissect from medial and lateral to the region of the soft triangle. Then the soft triangle is everted and the two edges of the dissection are joined under direct vision.

  ○ The posterior two thirds of the septum dissects the easiest and therefore, is a good place to start this dissection.

  ○ Always perform the dorsal reduction before the septoplasty to ensure 1 cm of septal cartilage will be left at the dorsal and caudal borders.

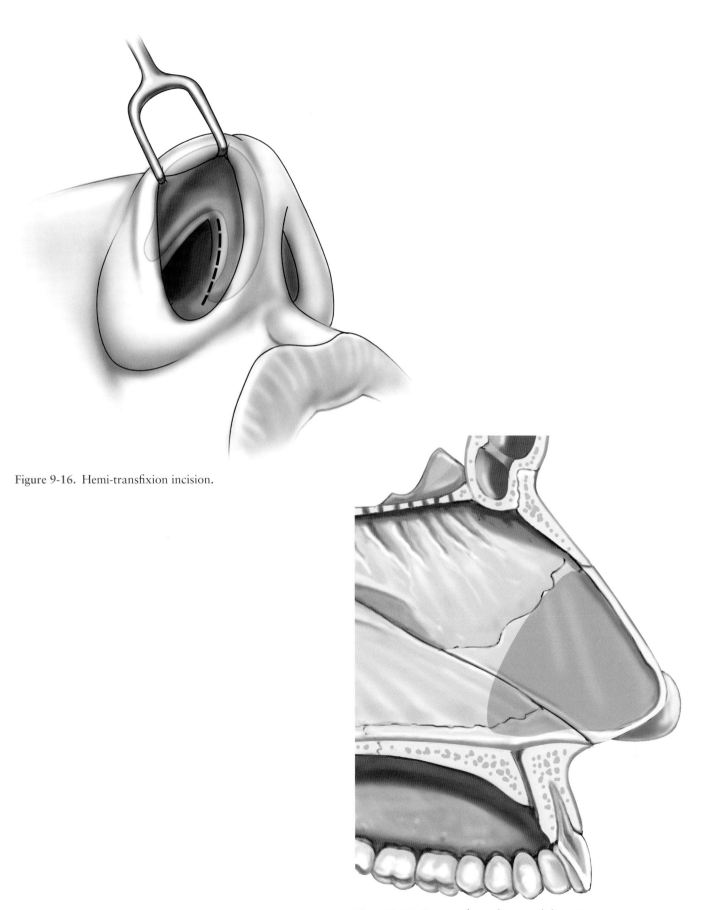

Figure 9-16. Hemi-transfixion incision.

Figure 9-17. Extent of septal mucosal dissection.

Chapter 10. Ear Cartilage Harvest

- *Indications*: The ear provides a readily accessible source of cartilage for structural support in the nose. Conchal cartilage is useful for support of the lateral sidewalls and alar rims (Figure 10-1). It can also be used for spreader grafts when septal cartilage is not available. It is noticeably less stiff and therefore more malleable than either septal or costal cartilage; however, both of these may be thinned to the appropriate thickness and pliability. If increased rigidity is necessary, ear cartilage may be reinforced with PDS foil that can be sutured to the graft. Composite skin and cartilage grafts can be harvested from the helical root for reconstruction of full thickness defects of the alar rim. Gentle scoring of the convex surface can create a roll of the cartilage to mimic the natural contour of the alar rim.

- *Markings*: Cartilage from the ear may be harvested from either an anterior or posterior approach with adequate camouflage of the incision. The posterior incision is marked as a curvilinear line over the middle of the posterior ear (Figure 10-2). The incision for an anterior approach is similarly placed at the superior margin of the conchal bowl below the antihelix. In harvesting cartilage from the conchal bowl, care must be taken to avoid destruction of the helical root as it merges with the conchal bowl (Figure 10-3). A large piece of conchal cartilage may be harvested in a kidney-bean shape to minimize distortion of conchal anatomy. Composite grafts of skin and cartilage should be taken from the proximal portion of the helical root where advancement of the distal end allows for primary closure. When a large piece of cartilage is desired, a posterior approach is used because of the loose subcutaneous areolar plane that facilitates dissection and exposure. However, when a skin-cartilage composite graft is necessary, often the anterior approach is preferable because of the tight attachment between the cartilage and anterior ear skin. When the posterior approach is used for a composite graft, the overlying skin is too mobile over the cartilage. The anterior approach is useful when harvesting composite grafts for correction of alar retraction.

- *Approach*: For a posterior approach, the skin incision is made with a scalpel and carried down to the level of the cartilage being careful not to incise the cartilage itself. Dissection over the cartilage proceeds with fine scissors within a relatively avascular plane to provide wide exposure. After double-checking the position of the planned resection from both anterior and posterior views, the scalpel is used to incise the cartilage itself. In doing so, a finger should be placed on the anterior aspect of the ear. The surgeon should feel a tactile "give" as the cartilage is split but before the skin has been cut. The finger adequately judges the depth of the incision so that skin over the contralateral surface is not violated. Obviously, one needs to be careful to avoid cutting one's finger with this maneuver. Once in the correct plane, a Freer elevator or tenotomy scissors can be used to dissect out the space on the opposite side of the cartilage. Further incision of the cartilage can then be performed under direct vision with either scissors or scalpel. The graft is removed and kept in moistened saline gauze until ready for use. Adequate hemostasis is achieved, the wound is irrigated, and the skin closed in a single layer.

- *Postoperative management*: A compressive dressing should be placed into and behind the conchal bowl to minimize fluid collection in the immediate postoperative period. A Vaseline-gauze dressing can be molded within the conchal bowl and placed behind the helical framework over the incision. On top of this a gentle dry gauze dressing should be wrapped around the head and left in place for 24 hours, at which time it may be changed and any subcutaneous blood identified. Alternatively, Xeroform™ gauze can be rolled into two small balls with one placed anterior to the harvest site and one posterior. A 3-0 Prolene mattress is then used for gentle compression of the skin—tight enough to approximate but loose enough not to strangulate. If a compressive dressing is not done, a hematoma is likely to develop, which may lead to cartilage destruction and a cauliflower ear deformity. The fluid may also serve as a nidus for infection.

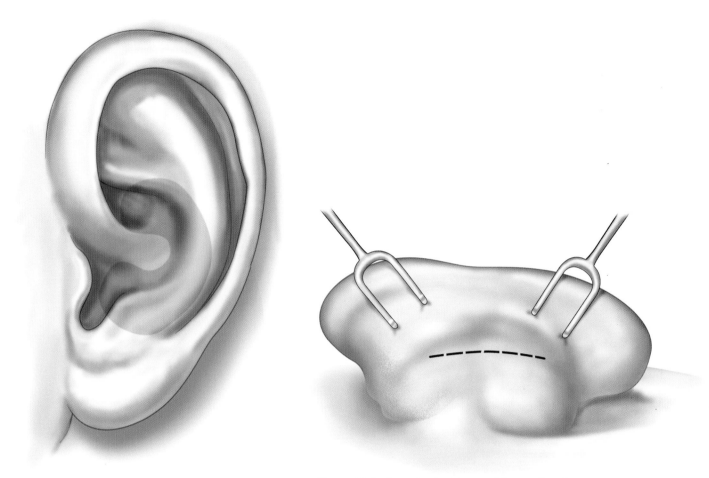

Figure 10-1. Extent of conchal cartilage harvest.

Figure 10-2. Posterior incision used for cartilage harvest.

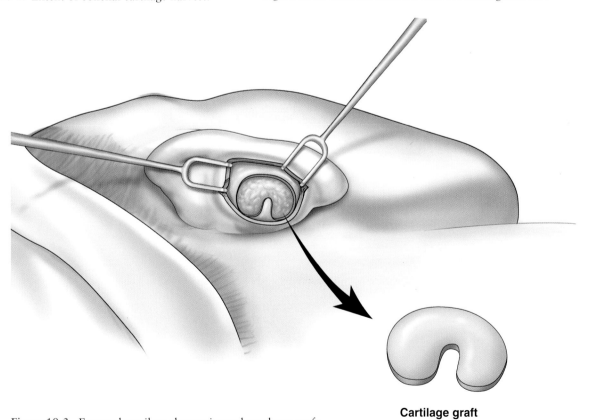

Cartilage graft

Figure 10-3. Exposed cartilage donor site and resultant graft.

- *Pitfalls*:
  - Proper anatomic definition of the conchal bowl will be lost if the helical root is resected during graft harvest. This key structure should be identified and marked preoperatively.
  - A postoperative gentle pressure dressing and close postoperative follow-up to evacuate any fluid is important.
- *Tips*:
  - The helical root should be identified and marked preoperatively. As such, cartilage graft harvested from the conchal bowl will assume a kidney-bean shape with a cutout from where the helical root is left in situ.
  - Do not crush ear cartilage to "smooth it out." Crushing leads to a pebbly, irregular appearance and may calcify.[1]

REFERENCE

1. Gruber R, Pardun J, Wall S. Grafting the nasal dorsum with tandem ear cartilage. *Plast Reconstr Surg.* 2003;112:1110.

Chapter 11. Calvarial Bone Harvest

- *Indications*: The calvarium provides an excellent donor source when bone is necessary for reconstruction. It may be safely harvested to reconstruct a nose with deficient structural support. The adult skull consists of outer and inner tables of dense cortical bone separated by the diploic space, a layer of cancellous bone. Either the full outer table of bone or a thinner shaving of the outer table can be safely obtained as graft material.

- *Markings*: Bone from the skull is best harvested from the flatter lateral areas of the parietal bone. Care should be taken not to harvest bone over the midline to avoid serious injury to the intracranial sagittal sinus. A gentle zig-zag incision is drawn parallel to the supraorbital neurovascular bundle to minimize postoperative paresthesia and visibility of the incision, especially when the hair is wet (Figure 11-1).

- *Approach*: The skin of the scalp does not need to be shaved prior to the incision but surgical lubrication is useful to keep the hair against the scalp. Liberal use of local anesthetic with epinephrine should be infiltrated and allowed time to work before beginning. The skin is incised with a scalpel and dissection proceeds down to the periosteum with electrocautery to minimize bleeding. The skin incision within the hair-bearing tissue can be beveled to minimize damage to the hair follicles and resultant postoperative scar alopecia. The desired amount of bone is outlined on the periosteum with the electrocautery.

- *Partial cortical harvest*: For thinner bone, the periosteum should be left intact so that it serves to hold smaller fragments of bone together. A wide, sharp osteotome is directed at the skull and advanced at roughly a 45-degree angle. The graft that is produced will fragment and tend to curl on itself but should be sufficient for areas where thin, non-weight-bearing bone is required.

- *Full cortical harvest*: To obtain a full table of calvarial bone, a thin channel is made with a fissure burr around the periphery of the area of bone desired (Figure 11-2). It is advisable to make sure the hair is lubricated and against the scalp and to use the shortest shaft possible on the drill. Additionally, a malleable retractor can be placed between the rotating drill shaft and the hair. The surgeon needs to be diligent to avoid getting loose hair caught in a rapidly spinning drill during this part of the harvest. The desired graft dimension is then outlined and drilled to the level of the diploic space. Careful inspection of the bony architecture will determine the appropriate depth. The diploic space tends to bleed more readily than the overlying cortical bone and visualization is easier when the bone is copiously irrigated while the surgeon is drilling. The posterior table of bone is left intact to prevent dural injury.

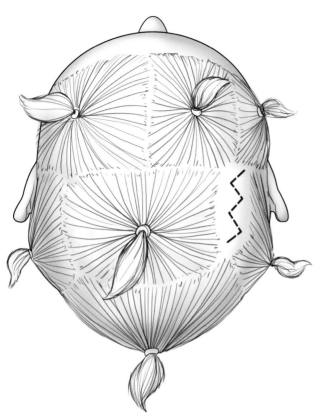

Figure 11-1. Location of a scalp incision for calvarial bone harvest.

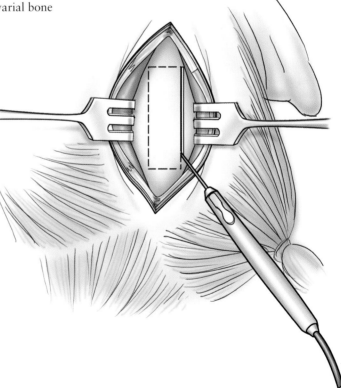

Figure 11-2. This image depicts incision through the periosteum of the calvarium with the electrocautery.

After the fissure burr has been used to outline the graft, a contouring burr is used along the outside edge of bone to create a bevel down to the interdiploic space (Figure 11-3). This bevel allows tangential placement of the osteotome during harvest, reducing the chance on intracranial exposure. The graft is carefully removed with a series of straight or curved osteotomes directed parallel to the surface of the bone to minimize penetration of the inner table (Figure 11-4).

Care should be taken to not over-chisel bone from one isolated area of the graft but rather advance the osteotome equally across all portions of the graft by moving the osteotome up and down the graft as harvest proceeds. This will minimize inadvertent fracture of the desired piece of bone. Care should also be taken to protect the graft from flying out of the operative field as the last connections to the diploic space are osteotomized. When the graft is removed, the underlying calvarial bone should be inspected and palpated for integrity of the posterior table (Figure 11-5). Hemostasis is achieved with either the electrocautery or a conservative amount of bone wax.

- *Inadvertent intracranial exposure*: Suspected violation of the posterior table and dural injury warrants wider exposure of the dura and primary repair of any lacerations. This should be done in concert with a neurosurgical colleague. The bone surrounding the accidental violation may be safely removed with a Kerrison rongeur or curette. It may be replaced once the dura is repaired with interrupted, braided 4-0 nylon sutures. Areas where the dura cannot be repaired primarily may require autogenous or alloplastic replacement material covered by hardening liquid sealant.
- *Closure*: A thin self-suctioning drain may or may not be used depending on the quality of the wound. The scalp is closed in layers: interrupted for the galea and either interrupted or running sutures for the skin. A running, locked suture will provide better hemostasis.

A standard pressure dressing around the head is added to minimize fluid collection beneath the scalp.

- *Postoperative management*: If a drain is left postoperatively, it can typically be removed the next day. The pressure dressing may be removed in the office at the first postoperative visit.
- *Pitfalls*:
  ○ The normal architecture of the adult skull may not be developed in younger patients and the individual cortices may be too thin in the elderly patient to warrant use of a calvarial bone graft in these populations.
  ○ Scar alopecia will result from injury to the subcutaneous follicles at the wound margins.
  ○ Injury to the underlying dura is of greater concern. Attempt to keep the angle of the osteotome tangential to the calvarium. Curved osteotomes that stay close to the underside of the outer cortex are helpful.
  ○ Bone grafts are prone to resorption and have a rigid feel.
- *Tips*:
  ○ A careful, beveled incision and generous use of local anesthetic with epinephrine to limit the need for electrocautery will minimize the risk of alopecia.
  ○ Aggressive cautery of the hair-bearing subcutaneous tissues should be avoided.
  ○ Care should be taken to adequately burr out the corners of the desired graft since these are areas where removal is commonly held up.
  ○ Place surgical lubricant in the hair at the periphery of the incision to keep it out of the way and thus minimize the chance of hair getting caught in the spinning drill.
  ○ The cutting edge of the osteotome should be kept as flat and as parallel as possible to the calvarial surface within the diploic space.
  ○ Bone wax may be used to control bleeding from the edges of the calvarium but it is a foreign body and its use should be minimized to reduce the risk of postoperative infection.

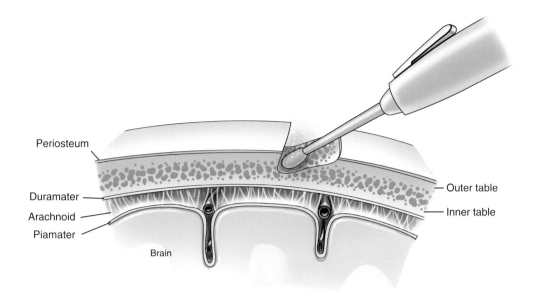

Periosteum

Duramater

Arachnoid

Piamater

Brain

Outer table

Inner table

Figure 11-3. Contouring burr to create a beveled edge down to the diploic space.

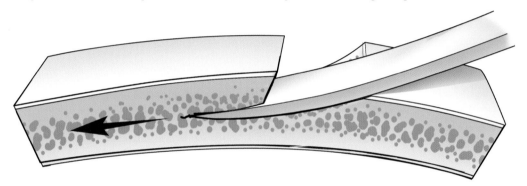

Figure 11-4. Horizontal direction of the osteotome.

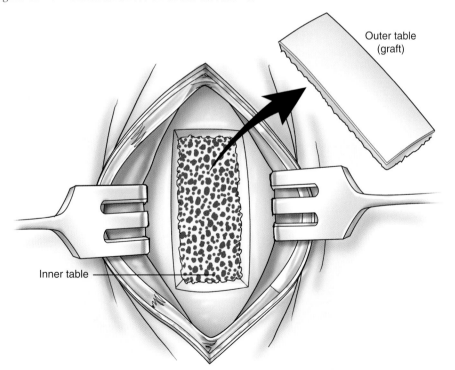

Outer table (graft)

Inner table

Figure 11-5. Removed outer table calvarial graft and resultant donor site.

Chapter 12. Costal Bone and Cartilage Harvest

- *Indications*: The rib is a useful graft donor site in that it allows the surgeon to harvest bone and cartilage through the same incision.
- *Markings*: The bone within the rib is found more laterally, while the cartilage is found more medially (Figure 12-1). The point where the transition occurs can generally not be appreciated by simple palpation over the skin. Any incision over the chest may be cheated medially or laterally to accommodate the surgeon's needs (primarily bone-lateral, primarily cartilage-medial). In women, an incision just inferior to the inframammary fold (IMF) allows access to the rib while preserving aesthetics; however, this location may need to be modified based on other factors. In men, the incision can be placed at the IMF as well or directly over the rib to be harvested. It is preferable to mark the length of the incision smaller than the desired graft length. The laxity of the chest skin allows the incision to be moved over the rib in all directions allowing dissection through a shorter incision. If necessary, the incision can always be lengthened.
- *Cartilage harvest approach*: The incision (about 5 cm in length) is made in the skin and carried down through the soft tissues to the periosteum of the ribs. Rectus muscle may be encountered and need to be divided or retracted medially before reaching the periosteum or perichondrium. The junction between the bone and cartilage may be identified by gently pressing a pointed cautery tip or #11 blade into the rib. The cartilaginous portion will be softer, the bony portion more brittle. A definite transition point should not be difficult to identify. Dissection should continue either medial or lateral to the transition point, depending upon the type of graft that is needed. Some surgeons prefer to leave the perichondrium on the cartilage and dissect in a plane just superficial to it, others prefer to dissect beneath the perichondrium. At one end of the dissection margin, the rib is carefully encircled, cognizant that the pleura is immediately adjacent to the undersurface of the rib (Figure 12-2). A needle tip set on 10-15 provides good exposure while cauterizing and keeping the dissection dry. This dissection begins at the superior and inferior edges of the rib and proceeds posteriorly toward the pleura for a distance about two-thirds the thickness of the rib. At this point, the surgeon should be at a safe distance from the pleura but should have a good view to initiate a dissection under the deep aspect of the rib with a periosteal elevator (Figure 12-3). Once the rib is circumferentially dissected, a Doyen retractor or malleable elevator is placed under the rib, and then a scalpel can be used to cut down on the rib while protecting the underlying pleura with a malleable retractor. After transection of the cartilage, the medial end can be gently lifted, exposing the tissue deep to the rib and allowing further dissection under direct vision.

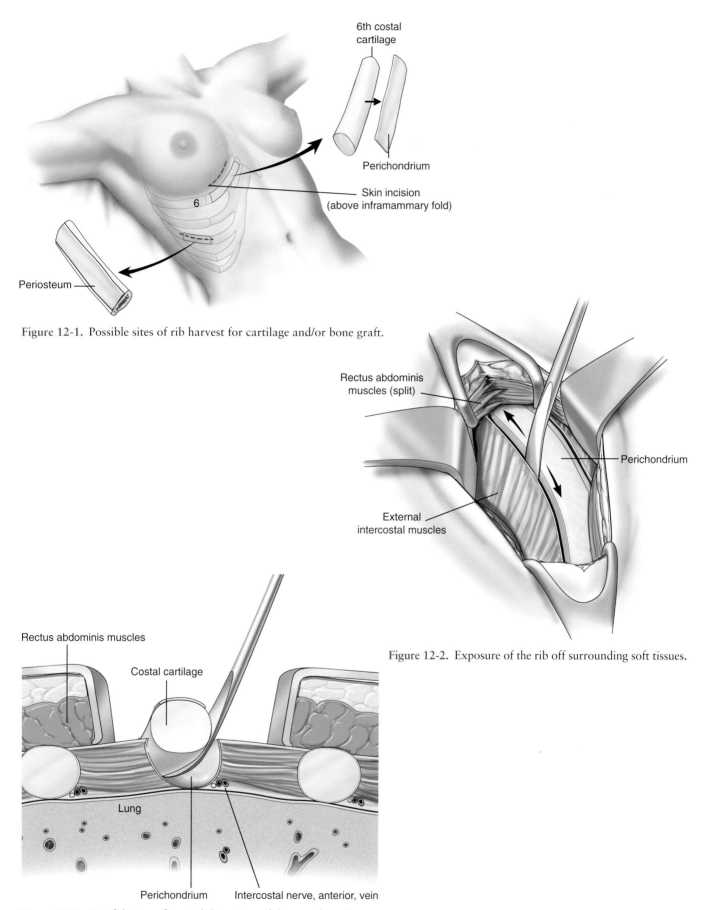

6th costal cartilage

Perichondrium

Skin incision
(above inframammary fold)

6

Periosteum

Figure 12-1. Possible sites of rib harvest for cartilage and/or bone graft.

Rectus abdominis
muscles (split)

Perichondrium

External
intercostal muscles

Figure 12-2. Exposure of the rib off surrounding soft tissues.

Rectus abdominis muscles

Costal cartilage

Lung

Perichondrium   Intercostal nerve, anterior, vein

Figure 12-3. Careful circumferential dissection of the costal cartilage.

- *Cartilage warping*: Cartilage grafts are prone to warping to various degrees. The extent and duration of active warping after harvest vary in the literature. However, some warping does occur and the majority occurs within the first hour after carving. Some basic principles can minimize the complications associated with cartilage warping. The perichondrium should be removed and the graft should be taken from a central portion of the rib. The straightest portion of the rib should be used and balanced carving should be done to equalize the intrinsic forces acting on the graft. Given that the majority of warping occurs within the first hour after manipulation, the graft should be carved early and set aside so that the degree and shape of the warping can be assessed prior to placement.[1,2,3]

- *Bone harvest approach*: The approach to the osseous rib is as above but slightly more lateral. After circumferential dissection of the osseous rib, the soft tissues may be further dissected laterally with a curved Doyen periosteal elevator. This is more effective for bone than it is for cartilage. The bony ends of the segment to be harvested may be cut with a saw or bone cutters but care should be taken to protect the deeper tissues with a malleable retractor. Once a free end is identified, it is helpful to place dry gauze around the end to pull the rib medially. This medial traction allows the Doyen elevator and the rib cutter to reach farther posteriorly facilitating harvest of adequate bone. Continuous irrigation is employed if a saw is used to cut the bone. There is no need to replace a single resected rib (or portion of cartilage) with filler material. Any divided muscle should be reapproximated and a drain can be left. The skin and soft tissues are closed in layers.

- *Pneumothorax*: Harvest should be careful to avoid injury to the underlying pleura and lung. Prior to closure, the wound should be filled with saline during a Valsalva maneuver and observed for air bubbles. An initial rush of bubbles may arise from trapped air pockets within the wound itself; however, a steady stream of bubbles indicates parenchymal damage to the lung requiring an indwelling chest tube. If no steady stream of air is detected but the pleura has been violated, any air will need to be removed from the pleural cavity. A small-gauge red rubber catheter is placed through the injured pleura and connected to suction to evacuate the air. The pleura is repaired around the catheter with a purse-string suture. While increasing inspiratory pressure from the ventilator (Valsalva maneuver), the catheter is removed as the suture is tightened. The wound may again be filled with saline or water and the presence of air noted.

- *Postoperative management*: A gauze and semiocclusive dressing can be placed over the incision. It is advisable to obtain a postoperative chest X-ray in the recovery room to identify the presence of any air in the pleural space. If the pleural cavity was inadvertently entered, the patient should be observed and serial chest X-rays obtained to either rule out or follow any postoperative pneumothorax.

- *Pitfalls*:
  - Dissect carefully around the rib to avoid injury to the pleura. Deeper dissection should be done under direct vision with the rib retracted out of the wound as much as possible.
  - Cartilage warping may occur weeks after placement compromising the symmetry of the final result.
  - If harvesting costochondral graft, take care to avoid injury to the costochondral junction.

- *Tips*:
  - The initial dissection of the rib should proceed on top of the rib to minimize bleeding from the costal vessels, which travel on the inferior aspect of the rib.
  - In a patient who has undergone previous rib harvest, one should use the same scar if there is a palpable rib within range of the incision.
  - Postoperative pain control may be achieved with a pain pump to deliver a continuous low dose of local anesthetic.
  - Older patients will have calcified cartilage, requiring a more medial dissection to obtain usable cartilage. A limited CT scan of the sternum with axial images (and coronal reformatting) of the sternum and costochondral junctions is useful in determining the degree and extent of chondral calcification.[4]
  - It is helpful to remove only the cartilage necessary for grafting. If the superior 75% is harvested leaving the inferior 25% intact, a contour deformity of the donor site can be minimized.
  - Leftover cartilage can be banked subcutaneously in the rib incision for future use. If the rib is not necessary for future surgery, it can be removed under local anesthesia in the office. If, however, it is necessary for a revision, the patient is spared a second painful rib harvest.

REFERENCES

1. Weber S, Cook TA, Wang TD. Irradiated costal cartilage in augmentation rhinoplasty. *Oper Techn Otolaryng.* 2007;18:274–283.
2. Adams W, Rohrich R, Gunter J, et al. The rate of warping in irradiated and nonirradiated homograft rib cartilage: A controlled comparison and clinical implications. *Plast Reconstr Surg.* 1999;103:265–270.
3. Gunter JP, Clark CP, Friedman R. Internal stabilization of autogenous rib grafts in rhinoplasty: A barrier to cartilage warping. *Plast Reconstr Surg.* 1997;100:161.
4. Marin VP, Landecker A, Gunter JP. Harvesting rib cartilage grafts for secondary rhinoplasty. *Plast Reconstr Surg.* 2008;121:1442.

Chapter 13. Iliac Crest Harvest

- *Indications*: The iliac crest provides adequate bone in patients who require a bone graft. The iliac crest is a bone donor site that can be used as an alternative to the cranium or the rib. It too has an inner cancellous marrow bounded on either side by cortical bone. Either the outer or inner tables of cortex can be harvested for grafting.
- *Neuroanatomy*: Care must be taken to avoid the lateral femoral cutaneous nerve, which innervates the skin of the lateral thigh. It exits the abdomen medial to the anterior superior iliac spine, deep to the inguinal ligament and in a groove between the sartorius and iliacus muscles. Injury to the nerve, called "Bernhardt syndrome," should be avoided at the time of iliac crest harvest. The ilioinguinal nerve runs between the external abdominal oblique and the internal abdominal oblique muscles at the level of the pelvic brim. It provides sensation to the root of the penis, scrotum, and anteromedial aspect of the thigh. It can be injured during harvest of the inner cortex of the iliac crest. Injury to the superior cluneal nerves has been reported at the time of posterior iliac crest bone harvest. The cutaneous superior cluneal nerves cross beneath the inguinal ligament in the lateral portion of the groin closer to the anterior superior iliac spine. As such, the incision is planned just lateral to the spine.
- *Approach*: The incision is marked 1 cm posterior from the anterior superior iliac spine to preserve the muscle attachments and minimize discomfort associated with their dissection (Figure 13-1). The incision is also 1 cm lateral to the iliac crest so that the final closure does not lie directly over this ridge of bone. The incision is made through the skin and carried down through the subcutaneous tissues. The periosteum over the iliac crest is reflected off the bone with an attempt made to keep it intact for later closure over the bone. The superior border of the crest may be preserved to minimize postoperative contour irregularity. A horizontal osteotomy is made ½ cm to 1 cm below the superior border

and two parallel osteotomies are made extending below this (Figure 13-2). The margins of the graft are completed with a lower horizontal osteotomy. The outer table of the iliac wing is then removed for graft material (Figure 13-3). Similarly, the inner table may also be used. If the inner table is chosen, care must be taken not to injure the pelvic structures, which lie medial to it. A Taylor retractor is useful at protecting the peritoneum while providing excellent vision of the medial cortex. After hemostasis is achieved, the wound is copiously irrigated, and a closed suction drain may be used. Fluff Avitene® placed in a bulb syringe can be blown into the harvest site for additional hemostasis. If spared, the periosteum over the defect may be repaired. The subcutaneous tissues and skin are then repaired in layers. A separate subcutaneous catheter may be left for infusion of anesthetic.

- *Postoperative management*: No specific care is needed in the postoperative period following iliac crest harvest. If a drain is used in the harvest site, it may be left until residual fluid output is minimal. Patients may be kept at bed rest for a day or two on account of the anticipated discomfort. Since there is no violation of the structural integrity of the hip joint, gentle range of motion may be resumed immediately after surgery.
- *Pitfalls*:
  - Change in sensation around the donor site is one of the most commonly reported complications of iliac crest bone harvest.
  - Bone grafts are prone to resorption and have a rigid feel.
- *Tips*:
  - Knowledge of the anatomy of the above mentioned nerves should be understood so that injury can be avoided.
  - Care should be used when harvesting the bone so that a usable piece of crest is available for contouring. Multiple fractures through the graft will result in a less-than-satisfactory segment for nasal support.

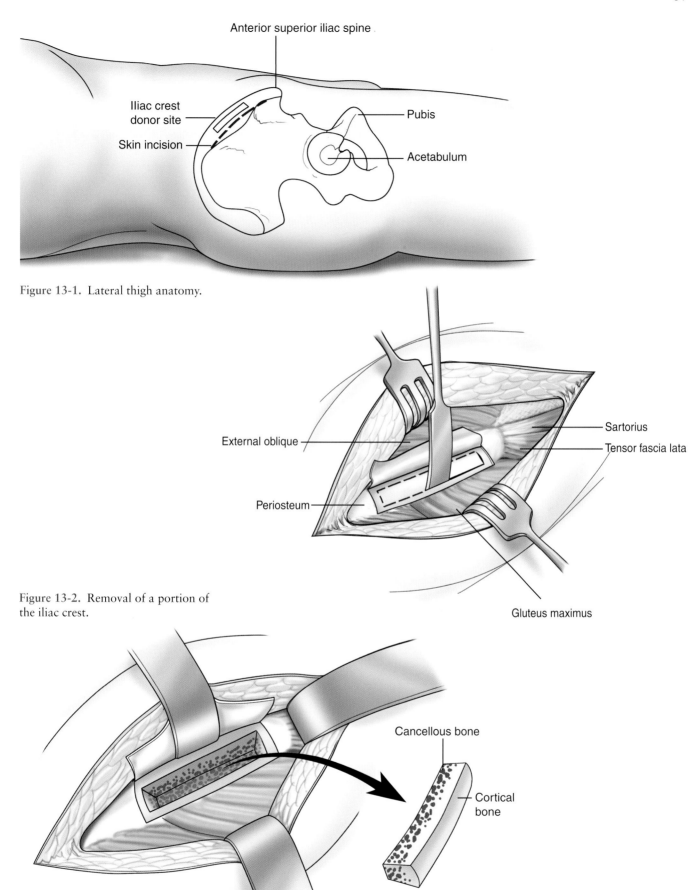

Figure 13-1. Lateral thigh anatomy.

Figure 13-2. Removal of a portion of the iliac crest.

Figure 13-3. Harvested outer table iliac crest cortical bone and the resultant donor site.

Chapter 14. Graft-depleted Patient

- *Indications*: There are five potential donor sites for autogenous tissue in secondary (or tertiary) rhinoplasty: ear cartilage, septal cartilage, rib cartilage, and calvarial and iliac bone. Patients who have exhausted the usual donor sites or were unhappy with prior donor procedures may require alternative options. Septal cartilage is optimal because it has strength and is planar, making it easy to shape into grafts that resist warping. Ear cartilage lacks structural support, and rib cartilage is prone to warping and painful as a donor site. Autogenous cartilage is the first choice; however, when supplies are depleted, other options are necessary.
- *Irradiated cartilage*: Irradiated cartilage is abundant and avoids a donor site. Some report that irradiated cartilage resorbs and is prone to warping even up to four weeks after carving.[1] However, the same study showed no difference in warping between irradiated and non-irradiated cartilage. Other studies have demonstrated long-term use with minimal resorption and acceptable warping characteristics.[2,3,4]
- *Polydioxanone flexible plate*: This is a resorbable polymer used primarily as a suture but now is FDA approved in various thicknesses of sheet form (Figure 14-1). Small pieces of cartilage that would be otherwise discarded can be approximated and sutured to the foil, creating a larger useable piece of graft material. Additionally, the foil can be used as a septal extension stabilizing strut when sutured to the dorsum and extending between the crura. The tip can be sutured to the foil to control projection and rotation.[5]
- *Bone*: In rare cases, bone has been used for indications that are traditionally treated with cartilage. Bone is prone to resorption, has a brittle feel, making it a less desirable graft material in most rhinoplasties. Cortical bone can be thinned and perforated to allow it to be used as a spreader graft in a cartilage depleted patient.[6]

REFERENCES

1. Adams W, Rohrich R, Gunter J, et al. The rate of warping in irradiated and nonirradiated homograft rib cartilage: A controlled comparison and clinical implications. *Plast Reconstr Surg.* 1999;103:265–270.
2. Weber S et al. Irradiated costal cartilage in augmentation rhinoplasty. *Oper Techn Otolaryng.* 2007;18:274–283.
3. Strauch B, Wallach SG. Reconstruction with irradiated homograft costal cartilage. *Plast Reconstr Surg.* 2003; 111:2405.
4. Lefkovits G. Nasal reconstruction with irradiated homograft costal cartilage. *Plast Reconstr Surg*—correspondence. 2004;113:1291.
5. Boenisch M, Mink A. Clinical and histological results of septoplasty with a resorbable implant. *Arch Otolaryngol Head and Neck Surg.* 2000;126:1373.
6. Prado A, Andrades P, Guerra C, Wisnia P. Cortical and partially cancellous bone spreader grafts: An alternative for the treatment of cartilage depleted noses. *Plast Reconstr Surg.* 2008;121:2136.

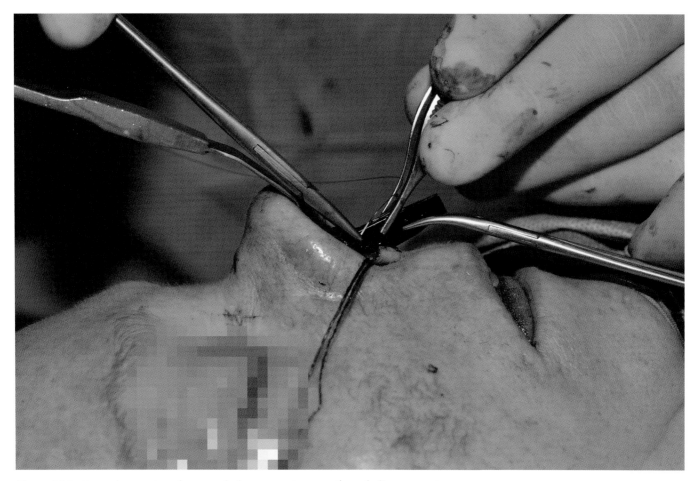

Figure 14-1. Lateral operative photograph demonstrating use of a polydioxanone sheet.

Chapter 15. Dorsal Hump Deformity

DEFINITION

The dorsal hump is typically noticed from the lateral view but requires analysis from all views (Figure 15-1). In general, a desirable dorsal profile for a male patient should be a fairly straight line from the radix to the tip. In women, a slight depression (about 2 mm) below this line with a distal depression before the tip ("supratip break") may be more appropriate. At its most superior aspect, the dorsum is made up of the paired nasal bones. More caudally, the dorsum is has a "T" shape composed of the midline septum and paired upper lateral cartilages. A dorsal hump may be due to excess nasal bone height, excess septal cartilage height, or most likely a combination of the two.

INDICATIONS

Patients with a "hump" or over-projecting dorsum are candidates for dorsal reduction. This may be performed as an isolated procedure or in conjunction with other maneuvers to reshape the nose.

It is important to assess the position of the radix preoperatively. A nose with an apparent "dorsal hump" that is actually due to a low radix may be better managed with dorsal augmentation between the hump and the radix to raise the radix to a more ideal position. The uneducated observer will miss the low position of the radix and reduce the dorsal lump in an attempt to better define the nasal tip. Dorsal reduction in this setting would severely compromise nasal aesthetics and be contraindicated.

MARKINGS

Some surgeons choose to mark the planned amount of reduction on the skin over the dorsum and refer to it as they incrementally reduce the bones and cartilages. The amount of reduction is based on the preoperative examination and 1:1 photographs. For patients undergoing an open approach, the incision across the columella may be marked preoperatively.

APPROACH

The dorsum may be approached via an open or closed technique depending on the surgeon's preference. However, isolated reduction of the dorsum will likely not require an open approach. With a closed approach, the dorsum may be exposed via an intercartilaginous incision. If an open approach is chosen, the columellar incision is made and carried around each nostril into bilateral infracartilaginous incisions inside the alar rim.

Once above the medial crura of the lower lateral cartilages, the tissues in the midline above the dorsal septum and nasal bones are dissected with scissors. It is important to establish a dissection plane just above the periosteum and perichondrium as the dissection proceeds. This helps to keep a dry field, maximizes soft issue over the dorsum to hide small irregularities, and minimizes tissue between the dissection and the dorsum. Inferiorly, the dorsal septum is identified and is mobile below its attachments to the upper lateral cartilage.

A small amount of lateral dissection is important to feather or contour the dorsum and prevent a flattened appearance. However, too aggressive lateral dissection should be avoided if nasal bone osteotomies are to be performed. Some soft tissue attachment should be left on the bones to hold them in place following infracture. A freely dissected nasal bone risks malposition after fracture. If dorsal resection is excessive, placement of spreader grafts (either free or folded from the medial edges of the upper lateral cartilages) should be considered.

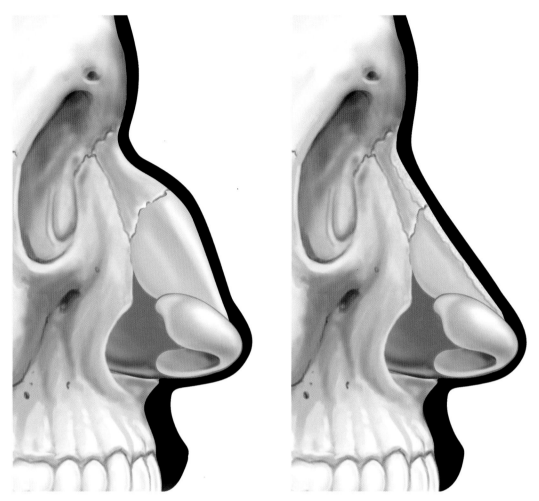

Figure 15-1. Dorsal hump deformity and its correction.

TECHNIQUE

Reduction of the dorsum is performed by separating it into its component parts, especially at the cartilaginous level where the upper lateral cartilages rest on the dorsal septum. Reduction of the bone is usually performed independent of the cartilage and may either precede or follow it.

The method for bony reduction depends on the amount of bone that will be removed (Figure 15-2). For smaller reductions, the bony dorsum may be taken down with rasps (Figure 15-3). A guarded osteotome is used when a larger amount of bone is to be removed (Figure 15-4). Care should be taken that the osteotome passes relatively superficially and does not create a divot in the radix. After the osteotome is used, rasps are used to smooth the dorsal contour. In addition to reducing and smoothing the central dorsum, the rasps should be oriented obliquely along the lateral edges to refine the dorsal aesthetic lines.

As the dorsum is incrementally resected, the skin should be frequently re-draped to confirm the adequacy of the reduction. A single suture may be used to temporarily close the columellar incision to accurately redrape the soft tissue envelope. A moistened finger is an excellent means of detecting subtle irregularities that may not be seen in the face of edema. Intraoperatively, the tip should project above the height of the dorsum to give a subtle supratip break. In thicker-skinned patients, this distance should be slightly greater. Once reduced, the dorsum should be inspected and palpated to identify the presence of an open roof. If present, osteotomy of the nasal bones must be performed to close the roof and re-create the pyramidal shape, which is addressed below.

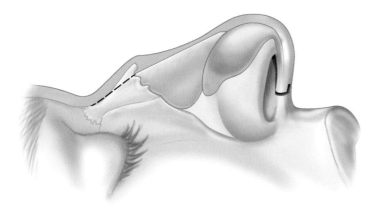

Figure 15-2. Planned reduction of the bony dorsum.

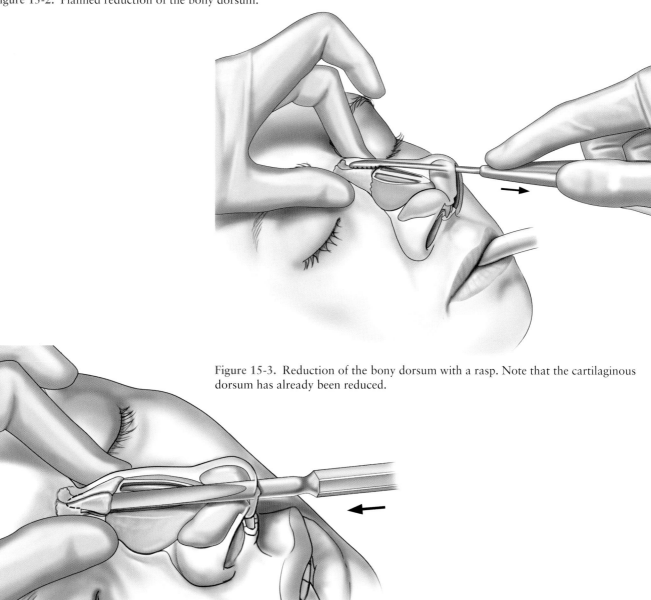

Figure 15-3. Reduction of the bony dorsum with a rasp. Note that the cartilaginous dorsum has already been reduced.

Figure 15-4. Reduction of the bony dorsum with an osteotome.

Once the bony dorsum has been addressed, a needle tip Bovie on a low setting or scalpel blade can be used to score the more inferior dorsal surface to identify a subperichondrial plane over the septum (Figure 15-5). The dorsal edge of the septum is gently grasped with a Brown-Adson forceps while a sharp Cottle elevator is used to start a subperichondrial dissection from an anteroposterior direction along the dorsal aspect of the septum. This can be tunneled proximally under the upper lateral cartilages, creating a subperichondrial tunnel (Figure 15-6). Once the tunnel has been established on both sides of the septum, a #15 scalpel blade can be placed adjacent to the septum, with the sharp edge facing upwards, and gently lifted to separate the upper lateral cartilages from the septum.[1,2] Once separated, the lateral cartilages will fall away from the midline septum.

Following separation of the caudal dorsum into the paired upper lateral cartilages and dorsal septum, reduction of the septal component is performed with either a scalpel or sharp scissors (Figure 15-7). For either, a Brown-Adson forceps can be used to grasp the more inferior septum for stability. If a scalpel is chosen, care must be taken not to injure the surrounding skin envelope. A #11 blade with the tip broken off is easy to use and the blunted tip minimizes the chance of inadvertent injury.

The medial edges of the upper lateral cartilages should be reduced separately to prevent over-resection. It is important to note that equal or less reduction of the upper lateral cartilages with respect to the septum should be performed so as to create a natural curvature of the dorsum. Excessive resection of the upper lateral cartilage will result in an inverted-V deformity. This occurs not infrequently because as the assistant pulls on the dorsal skin with a retractor to create space for adequate visualization, the freed upper lateral cartilages are pulled superiorly and anteriorly into a more artificial position (Figure 15-8). Resection of what may seem conservative may actually be excessive with the cartilage in this position. Excessive resection leads to a functional internal valve collapse and the unnatural inverted-V deformity. Following appropriate trimming, the upper lateral cartilages should be sutured back to the septal cartilage to reestablish structure and support. The subperiosteal pocket should then be irrigated with saline to evacuate any remaining fragments of bone and/or cartilage. The columellar incision is closed temporarily with a single subcutaneous suture to gauge the smoothness of the dorsum again with a moistened finger.

POSTOPERATIVE MANAGEMENT

Strips of ¼-in paper tape or surgical strips may be used to minimize the development of edema and minimize dead space after the dorsum has been reduced. An external splint may or may not be used.

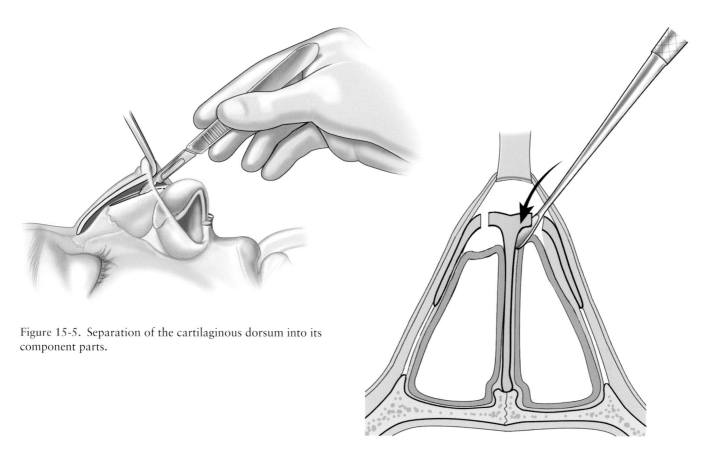

Figure 15-5. Separation of the cartilaginous dorsum into its component parts.

Figure 15-6. Creation of bilateral submucosal tunnel.

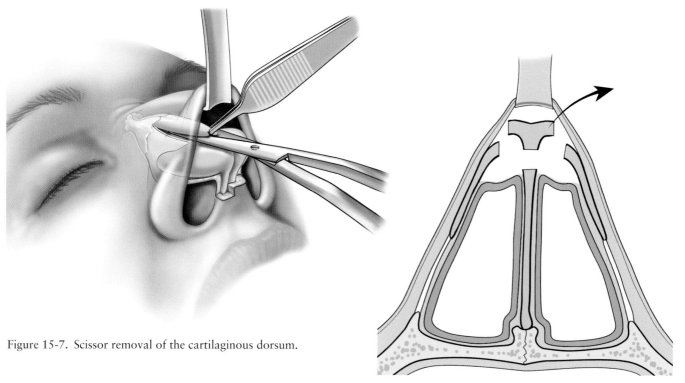

Figure 15-7. Scissor removal of the cartilaginous dorsum.

Figure 15-8. Removal of the cartilaginous dorsum and the upper lateral cartilages pulled into a falsely superior position due to the retractor.

PITFALLS

Reduction of the nasal dorsum may result in obvious complications, notably irregularity, overcorrection, or under-correction.

- Under-reduction results in a relative persistence of the deformity. Lateral examination of the dorsum during reduction will minimize the incidence of leaving the dorsum under-reduced. Under-resection is treated by additional reduction of either bone, cartilage, or both.
- Upper lateral cartilage injury/avulsion can occur with aggressive rasping along a straight line. This potential problem can be minimized by orienting the rasp in a slightly more oblique angle.
- Open roof deformity results from reduction of enough bone to expose the three components of the bony pyramid. An open roof deformity is best managed with lateral osteotomy of the nasal bones to close the opening. If too much dorsal bone is removed, a portion of it can also be replaced as a graft to cover the roof and more naturally round off the dorsum.
- An inverted-V deformity results from collapse at the level of the internal nasal valve. The stability of the upper cartilaginous vault depends not only on bony vault width but also on the height and width of the septum and upper lateral cartilages that comprise the roof.[4,5] Resection of that portion of the roof that contains the confluence of all three structures destabilizes the position of the upper lateral cartilages, allowing them to slide medially. This compromises airflow at the internal valves. The reduction in airflow may be avoided by recognition of the deformity and placement of dorsal and spreader grafts to maintain support. Conservative reduction of the upper lateral cartilage is advised.
- *Supratip deformity*: A supratip deformity, also known as a Pollybeak deformity, is postoperative fullness of the dorsum just above the tip. The etiologies of the supratip deformity are over-resection of the caudal dorsal septum, inadequate resection of the dorsal caudal septum, inadequate resection of cephalic lower lateral cartilages, and/or inadequate tip projection. Over-resection of the septum leads to a dead space that fills with blood and evolves into fibrous tissue creating undesired fullness in the supratip region. In order to minimize the dead space, taping is performed under the splint postoperatively. Additionally, a supratip suture can be placed. During the operation, the skin is temporarily closed and the region of the supratip break is marked with methylene blue through the skin to the underlying cartilage. The nose is opened again and a suture is placed from the deep dermis to the underlying cartilage where indicated by the methylene blue staining. This suture helps in minimizing dead space. An angiocatheter is also used at the end of the case to irrigate any residual blood prior to final splint application. Inadequate cephalic trim of the lower lateral cartilages will cause supratip fullness and is treated by further resection. If a supratip deformity is noted postoperatively, initial treatment during the first 4 weeks is taping. If there is no response by 6 to 8 weeks postoperatively, deep steroid injections can be used (0.2 cc to 0.4 cc of 20 mg/cc triamcinolone). If after 1 year there is a persistent deformity, surgical correction can be performed.[3]
- Inadequate tip projection results in a tip that is too low giving the illusion of a supratip deformity, yet when the tip is placed at the ideal position, the supratip deformity is corrected.
- Dorsal hump reduction will make the nose look wider and potentially increase cephalic tip rotation. Nasal osteotomies should be considered when dorsal hump reduction is performed.
- *Saddle nose deformity*: Over-reduction of the dorsum will result in low dorsal height and a drastically concave appearance on lateral view. This is commonly referred to as a "saddle nose deformity." It might also produce an open roof deformity at the confluence of the nasal bones and septum. Reducing the dorsum in small increments and checking the height after each attempt is the best method to prevent excessive resection. This is best done with a rasp rather than an osteotome, especially as one is getting comfortable with rhinoplasty surgery. If over-resection is noted at the time of the primary rhinoplasty, correction involves replacement of a portion of the resected tissue back onto the dorsum with either internal or external stabilization. Tape over the skin with a moldable splint will allow the tissue to heal back to the dorsum. Secondary reconstruction of the saddle nose deformity involves the addition of replacement material to augment the dorsum (see dorsal augmentation, chapter 16). Autogenous choices include cartilage, bone, or fascia. Sources of bone include the ribs, calvarium, or iliac crest. Sources of cartilage include the ribs, ear, or nasal septum. The replacement material should be positioned from the superior-most point of recession to the supratip area. The middle crura of the lower lateral cartilages should project above the level of the material to create a smooth transition and a slight supratip break.
- *Dimensional interplay*: Reduction of the dorsum affects other regions of the nose that must be considered. The dorsal aesthetic lines may be altered requiring spreader grafts to restore the dorsal nasal roof. Reduction of the nasal pyramid may create a nasal trapezoid giving the dorsum a wider appearance requiring nasal osteotomies to narrow for aesthetics or to close an open roof. If the hump has been removed and the dorsum narrowed, there is a good chance that the tip will now need to be refined and narrowed to bring it back into harmony with the new dimensions of the dorsum. Dorsal reduction may also affect the length of the nose, position of the columella, contour of the

nostrils, size of the alar base, and the internal nasal valves.[6,7,8]

TIPS

- The presence of a low radix should be identified preoperatively. This will minimize the chance of further reducing an already low dorsum. In such patients, the dorsum should be raised either segmentally or entirely and the amount of tip reduction should be limited.[6]
- To minimize the possibility of internal nasal valve collapse, the upper lateral cartilages should be maximally preserved.
- When combining a dorsal reduction with a septoplasty, the dorsal reduction should be performed first. This assures that 1 cm of dorsal and caudal septal cartilage will be preserved.
- When sufficient upper lateral cartilage is present at its medial edge, it can be reflected inward and serve as an autospreader graft to minimize the chance of internal valve collapse.
- Injection of corticosteroids is not indicated for any type of supratip deformity for several months after the primary rhinoplasty.

REFERENCES

1. Ponsky D, Eshraghi Y, Guyuron B. The frequency of surgical maneuvers during open rhinoplasty. *Plast Reconstr Surg.* 2010 Jul;126(1):240–244.
2. Rohrich RJ, Muzaffar AR, Janis JE. Component dorsal hump reduction: The importance of maintaining dorsal aesthetic lines in rhinoplasty. *Plast Reconstr Surg.* 2004 Oct;114(5):1298–1308.
3. Guyuron B, DeLuca L, Lash R. Supratip deformity: A closer look. *Plast Reconstr Surg.* 2000;105:1140.
4. Sheen, JH. Spreader graft: A method of reconstructing the roof of the middle nasal vault following rhinoplasty. *Plast Reconstr Surg.* 1984;73:230.
5. Constantian MB, Clardy RB. The relative importance of septal and nasal valvular surgery in correcting airway obstruction in primary and secondary rhinoplasty. *Plast Reconstr Surg.* 1996;98:38.
6. Constantian MB. Four common anatomic variants that predispose to unfavorable rhinoplasty results: A study based on 150 consecutive secondary rhinoplasties. *Plast Reconstr Surg.* 2000 Jan;105(1):316–331; discussion 332–333.
7. Constantian MB. Distant effects of dorsal and tip grafting in rhinoplasty. *Plast Reconstr Surg.* 1992;90:405.
8. Constantian MB. An alternate strategy for reducing the large nasal base. *Plast Reconstr Surg.* 1989;83:41.

Chapter 16. Dorsal Augmentation

- *Indications*: Patients who lack adequate height of the bony and/or cartilaginous dorsum may require dorsal augmentation (Figure 16-1). In general, a desirable dorsum for a male patient should be a fairly straight line from the radix to the tip. In women, a slight depression (about 2 mm) below this line (supratip break) may be more appropriate. A "saddle nose deformity" might be a consequence of prior trauma, including necrosis of the supporting septal cartilage secondary to cocaine use. Management requires the addition of supporting material to reconstruct the deficient framework and re-elevate the depressed soft tissues. Historically, a number of replacement materials have been described, but the authors strongly prefer autogenous tissue. Autogenous tissue offers greater resistance to infection than alloplastic material, which is prone to infection and extrusion long term. Cartilage provides a good replacement material since it is autogenous and readily available from the septum, ears, and ribs. In patients who are graft depleted or require greater elevation, bone graft from variable sources (rib, calvarium, iliac crest) can be used. Generally, cartilage is preferred over bone because the latter is hard, brittle, and prone to resorption. In the absence of adequate tissue and/or the desire to avoid donor site morbidity, biocompatible alloplastic materials, such as polyethylene and polytetrafluoroethylene (PTFE), have been utilized.[1,2] The choice of implant is at the discretion of the surgeon and should be based primarily on patient safety.

- *Markings*: No specific markings are required, although the relative contributions of the nasal bones and the septal and upper lateral cartilages should be identified preoperatively. The specific area of deficiency and a rough estimate of the boundaries of the soft tissue pocket should also be noted. External incisions for an open approach are similar to those described previously.

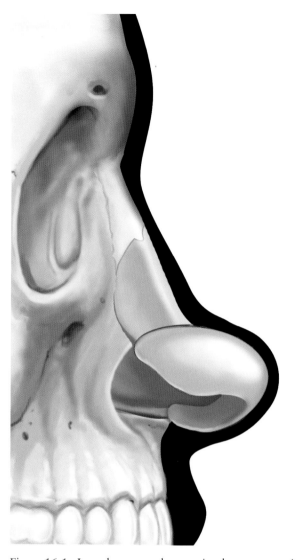

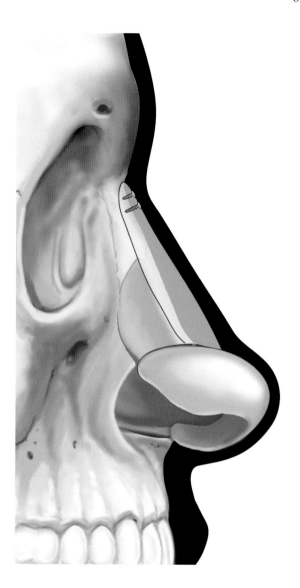

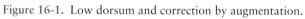

Figure 16-1. Low dorsum and correction by augmentation.

- *Approach*: Modification of the dorsum may be performed via an open or an endonasal approach, but in order to visualize the recipient bed, an open approach is recommended (Figure 16-2). In either the open or closed approach, scissor dissection then proceeds over the septum to the radix. (Figure 16-3). The soft tissue pocket over the dorsum should be made just wide enough to facilitate placement of the graft but not wide enough to permit undesirable malposition. The dorsal aspect of the nose should be sufficiently rasped to create an osseocartilaginous surface to which the graft can incorporate.
- *Several options for graft replacement exist:*
  - *Septal cartilage*: Septal cartilage may be used for augmentation up to 2 mm. However, septal cartilage is frequently used for other grafts or is unavailable. When available, it is easily harvested through a septoplasty approach. It can then be shaped and sutured into its desired position.[3]
  - *Ear cartilage*: For a deficiency of 3–6 mm, ear cartilage is an option. It is easily harvested and its use allows any available septum to be used for other grafts. If the cavum concha and cymba concha are harvested, a straight piece of cartilage can be harvested and smaller pieces can be sutured to the larger piece. If curvature of the ear cartilage is a problem, a polydioxanone foil can serve as a rigid platform to both flatten the ear cartilage as well as serve as a base to which multiple pieces of cartilage can be sutured.[4]
  - *Rib cartilage*: Rib cartilage can be harvested in a multitude of dimensions and is generally abundant in younger and middle-aged patients. There may be some calcification in older patients, and a CT scan can be obtained to identify this calcification preoperatively. The rib is harvested as described above (Chapter 12) and is then carved into the proper dimension. The graft should be shaped like a kayak, narrow cephalically and caudally with its widest dimension at the location of the osseocartilaginous vault. The major problem with rib cartilage is warping. A K-wire can be placed in the graft to resist this tendency. It is recommended to carve the general shape of the graft, then place the K-wire before proceeding to final dimensional detailing. Occasionally,

a small detailed graft can fracture during K-wire placement, so it is preferable to place the wire while the graft still has some bulk.
  - *Costochondral graft*: When a large volume of material is necessary from the radix to the tip, a costochondral graft is very useful. Its proximal portion is bone so it will hold a fixation screw and fuse to the underlying nasal bones. The distal portion is cartilage and will have the natural consistency of the distal two thirds of the cartilaginous nose. Because it is congruous with the bony portion, warping is decreased. Because of the larger size of this graft, it is recommended to deepen the radix so the proximal portion of the graft does not compromise the nasofrontal angle. This graft may also be attached to a columellar strut for more support if indicated.[5]
  - *Diced cartilage*: Cartilage from any site can be harvested and minced into 0.5-mm to 1.0-mm particles, which are stored in dilute antibiotic solution. The minced cartilage is then placed in fascia harvested from the temporalis through a hair-bearing incision. The fascia is sutured into a tube and the cartilage is injected into the fascia with a 1-cc syringe with the tip cut off. This then becomes a tube of fascia-filled cartilage that is inserted into the dorsal pocket. Particulate cartilage can also be injected around rib grafts to smooth the edges. Neither of these methods is prone to resorption, but the uncovered grafts may become palpable or visible. It is not recommended to wrap the cartilage in Surgicel® because its use has shown to increase cartilage resorption. This technique works well in that any cartilage source can be used and allows use of any leftover cartilage. Warping is not a concern, and the fascial cartilage complex can actually be molded for 10 to 14 days after the operation to maintain ideal dimensions.[6,7]
  - *Irradiated chondral cartilage*: Irradiated cartilage is abundant and avoids a donor site. Some authors report that irradiated cartilage resorbs and is prone to warping even up to 4 weeks after carving.[8] However, the same study showed no difference in warping between irradiated and nonirradiated cartilage. Other studies have demonstrated long term use with minimal resorption and acceptable warping characteristics.[9,10,11]

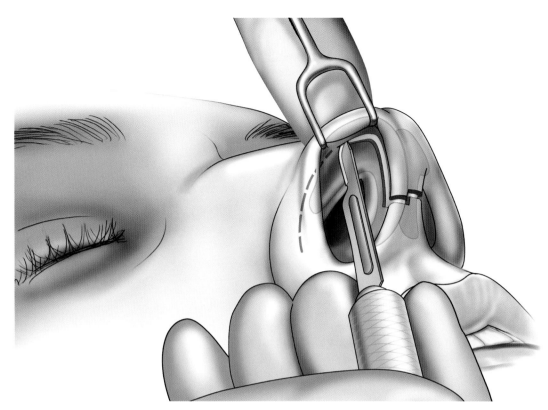

Figure 16-2. Approach to the dorsum via a transcolumellar incision.

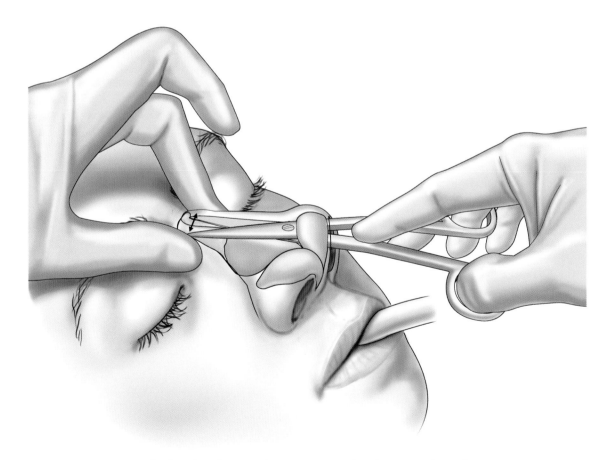

Figure 16-3. Creation of a dorsal pocket just above periosteum for placement of a graft.

- *Technique:*
  - *Graft contouring*: Following harvest, the graft can be manipulated by cutting it or contouring it with a scalpel or burr to the desired size. Fine rhinoplasty files are also useful in smoothing and contouring grafts. A concavity may be created on the inferior surface to stabilize the graft and maximize contact to the underlying dorsum. The edges can be beveled to allow the graft to better blend into the surrounding soft tissues (Figure 16-4). Several pieces of cartilage can also be stacked to create greater height.
  - *Graft placement*: The graft can be guided into place with a transcutaneous suture tied over a bolster and removed after 1 to 2 weeks. The suture is started through the skin just superior to the pocket for the graft and retrieved through the access incision. Suture on a straight needle works well for this purpose. It is passed through the skin, then through the graft, and then again supraperiosteally back up the dorsum and out of the skin just lateral to the opposite end of the suture. It is tied over a bolster of petroleum gauze for fixation. If any irregularity is palpable or visible after graft placement, the graft can be removed and modified or minor irregularities may be covered with small pieces of fascia. Occasionally, a piece of AlloDerm™ may be placed over the dorsum to smooth the final contour.
  - *Graft fixation*: Additional fixation of the graft can be performed in any of several ways.[12] The least invasive is a simple external tape dressing over the skin. While not the most secure option, it will hold the graft in place if the pocket offers little mobility. Temporary fixation of the graft to underlying bone can be performed with either one or two K-wires or one or two titanium screws. The K-wires are passed percutaneously into graft and into the underlying frontal bone being careful not to pass the tip too far. A small-gauge 8-mm or 10-mm length screw can also be placed through a small vertical incision in the region of the glabella over the superior portion of an osseous graft (Figures 16-5 and 16-6). The incision does not have to be long and will usually heal without a perceptible scar. A hole is drilled through the graft and into the underlying bone. The screw is then placed along the same trajectory without directly visualizing the hole. A second screw may be placed through the same incision and into the graft slightly inferior to the first.
  - *Postoperative management*: A splint of either plaster or moldable plastic should be placed over a standard tape dressing over the dorsum. It is kept in place for approximately 2 weeks to allow for healing of soft tissue around the graft.
- *Pitfalls*:
  - Grafts of cartilage may be placed either too low or too high in relation to the glabella and nasion.
  - Postoperatively, the graft may also migrate if dissection of the pocket is too extensive.
  - Dorsal augmentation may make the nose look narrower and cause the tip to rotate inferiorly. The tip may need a tip rotation suture after dorsal augmentation.
- *Tips*:
  - Dissection of the pocket should be directly over the bone to minimize any soft tissue between the graft and the underlying bone and to maximize the blood supply of the skin flap over the graft.
  - The pocket for the graft should be limited to the size of the graft to minimize the risk of malposition.
  - The edges of the graft, whether cartilage, bone, or alloplast, should be "softened" by beveling so that they taper into the surrounding nasal sidewalls and soft tissues. Sharp edges will be seen especially beneath a thin skin envelope.
  - A suture may be anchored to the end of the graft, brought through the skin in the region of the nasion, and tied over a bolster to help position the graft and minimize postoperative malposition.

REFERENCES

1. Sajjadian A, Naghshineh N, Rubinstein R. Current status of grafts and implants in rhinoplasty: Part II. Homologous grafts and allogenic implants. *Plast Reconstr Surg.* 2010; 125(3):99e–109e.
2. Peled Z, Warren A, Johnston P. The use of alloplastic materials in rhinoplasty surgery: A meta-analysis. *Plast Reconstr Surg.* 2008;121:85–92.
3. Gunter J, Rohrich R. Augmentation rhinoplasty: Dorsal onlay grafting using shaped autogenous septal cartilage. *Plast Reconstr Surg.* 1990;86:39.
4. Gruber R, Pardun J, Wall S. Grafting the nasal dorsum with tandem ear cartilage. *Plast Reconstr Surg.* 2003;112:1110.
5. Daniel R. Rhinoplasty and rib grafts: Evolving a flexible operative technique. *Plast Reconstr Surg.* 1994;94:597.
6. Daniel RK, Calvert J. Diced cartilage grafts in rhinoplasty surgery. *Plast Reconstr Surg.* 2004;113:2156.
7. Erol O. The Turkish delight: A pliable graft for rhinoplasty. *Plast Reconstr Surg.* 2000;105:1838.
8. Adams W, Rohrich R, Gunter J et al. The rate of warping in irradiated and nonirradiated homograft rib cartilage: A controlled comparison and clinical implications. *Plast Reconstr Surg.* 1999;103:265–270.
9. Weber S et al. Irradiated costal cartilage in augmentation rhinoplasty. *Oper Techn Otolaryng.* 2007;18:274–283.
10. Strauch B, Wallach SG. Reconstruction with irradiated homograft costal cartilage. *Plast Reconstr Surg.* 2003; 111:2405.
11. Lefkovits G. Nasal reconstruction with irradiated homograft costal cartilage. *Plast Reconstr Surg.*—correspondence. 2004;113:1291.
12. Gunter JP, Clark CP, Friedman RM. Internal stabilization of autogenous rib cartilage grafts in rhinoplasty: A barrier to cartilage warping. *Plast Reconstr Surg.* 1997;100:161–169.

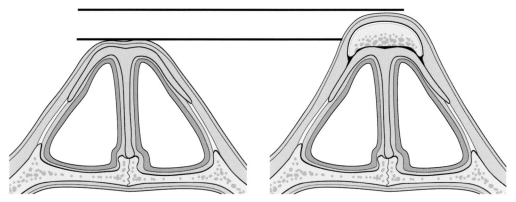

Figure 16-4. Augmentation of the dorsum with a graft. Note the slightly hollowed undersurface of the graft to minimize mobility and maximize surface contact.

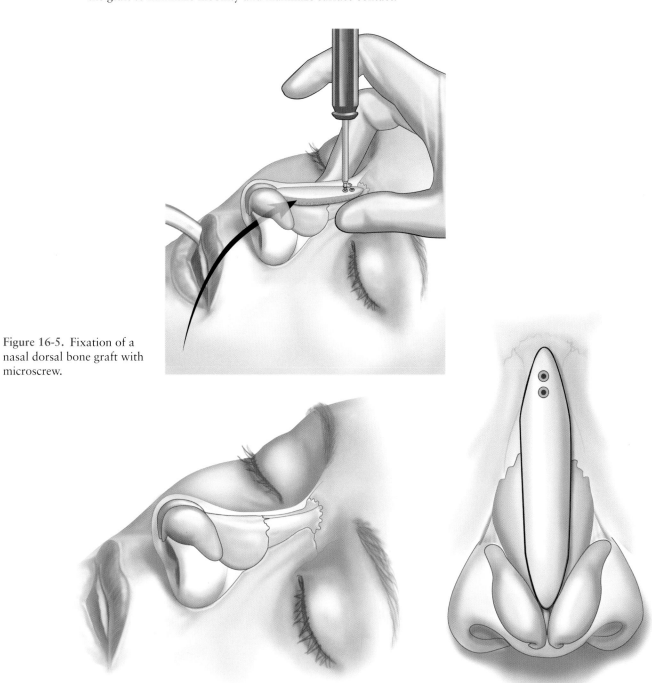

Figure 16-5. Fixation of a nasal dorsal bone graft with microscrew.

Figure 16-6. Dorsal graft in place, fixed at the radix and covered distally by the lower lateral cartilages.

Chapter 17. Radix Reduction

- Patients with excessive anterior protrusion of the nasal bones in the area of the nasion are candidates for reduction of the radix (Figure 17-1).
- *Markings*: No specific markings are required; however, a rough estimate of the amount of reduction required should be decided.
- *Approach*: A variety of incisions may be used to approach the radix. Via an open approach, the radix may be accessed via a columellar incision and standard dissection over the lower lateral cartilages and dorsum. Using a closed technique, an intranasal intercartilaginous incision extended along the caudal aspect of the cartilaginous septum may be used to expose the dorsum.
- *Technique*: Dissection proceeds along the dorsal midline with a scissors. At the level of the nasal bones, a Freer or key elevator may be used to dissect in a subperiosteal plane. The bony prominence at the nasofrontal angle may then be reduced using a variety of rasps or, if available, a guarded burr, which is exposed only at its inferior, cutting aspect[1] (Figure 17-2). Often, a curved rasp mirrors the natural anatomy of the radix and provides the most controlled, efficacious reduction (Figure 17-3). Bone may also be removed with a Lempert rongeur to address the most superior aspects of the radix. At the conclusion of the reduction, the soft tissue pocket should be irrigated with sterile saline to remove any loose bone or soft tissue and then combined with other procedures on the nose if indicated. Closure is performed in the standard fashion.
- Radix reduction at the superior (cephalad) portion of the nose will increase nasal length because it moves the nasion superiorly.
- Postoperatively, a tape dressing beneath a molded plastic or plaster splint over the entire dorsum may be used to minimize edema over the area of resection and maintain contour.
- *Pitfalls*:
  - Because several muscles run through the region of the radix, bleeding in an area difficult to directly visualize may occur with vigorous dissection.
  - If additional lateral osteotomies of the nasal bones are planned, care should be taken to preserve some lateral attachments of soft tissue to the nasal bones so that the osteotomies do not leave free-floating fragments of bone.
  - Conservative reduction of the radix, which is safe, often does not achieve noticeable diminution in the anterior projection of the overlying soft tissue. More aggressive reduction, however, may lead to violation of the frontal sinus, injury to the underlying mucosa, or over-reduction.
  - Radix reduction may give the illusion of increased intercanthal distance and may increase nasal length.
- *Tips*:
  - Adequate infiltration of the radix with local anesthetic with epinephrine and allowing sufficient time to elapse between injection and manipulation will minimize bleeding during dissection.
  - The patient should also be aware that the amount of soft tissue reduction does not follow the bone in an equal amount and that the amount of reduction is ultimately limited.

REFERENCE

1. Guyuron B. Guarded burr for deepening of the nasofrontal junction. *Plast Reconstr Surg.* 1989;84:513.

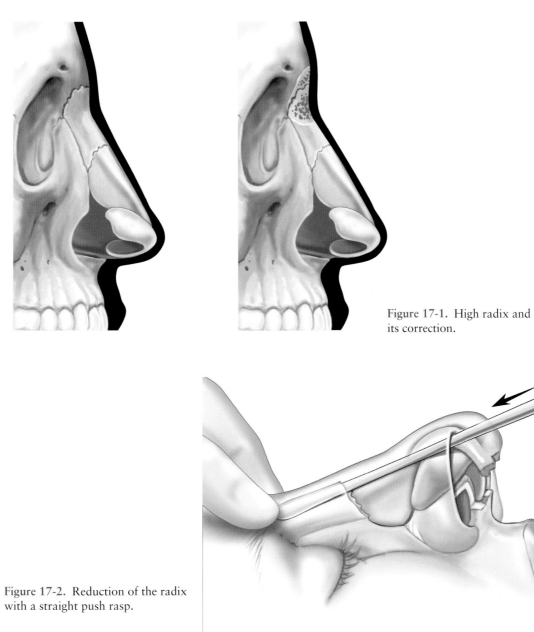

Figure 17-1. High radix and its correction.

Figure 17-2. Reduction of the radix with a straight push rasp.

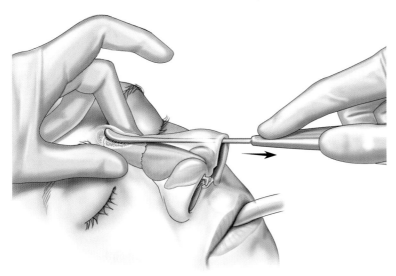

Figure 17-3. Schematic drawing depicting reduction of the radix with a curved pull rasp.

Chapter 18. Radix Augmentation

- Hollowing in the area of the radix is not an uncommon concern. Radix grafts are used to augment a deficient nasofrontal angle or move the radix breakpoint superiorly (Figure 18-1). A low radix may contribute to the appearance of a short nose, and improvement is achieved by augmentation of the radix.
- On a lateral photograph of the patient, the surgeon should make an estimate of the amount of correction needed. No specific markings are required; however, the area planned for the subcutaneous pocket of the graft may be outlined on the skin. The eventual height of the radix will need to be determined on the table.
- Creation of a pocket in the region of the radix is via dissection over the dorsum. The dorsum may be approached by an endonasal or open nasal approach. Via the open approach, the radix is accessed via a columellar skin incision and standard dissection over the lower lateral cartilages and dorsum. Using the closed technique, an intranasal intercartilaginous incision extended along the caudal aspect of the cartilaginous septum may be used to expose the dorsum. A scissors is used to take the soft tissue off the underlying dorsum. At the level of the radix, a Freer elevator is used to complete the dissection in a subperiosteal plane. The soft tissue pocket should be irrigated with sterile saline prior to placement of a graft to remove any loose fragments.
- Augmentation of the radix may be performed with autogenous or alloplastic material. Autogenous material is recommended and can be obtained from one of several sources including the septum, rib, or ear. Septal cartilage serves as an ideal graft material if it is available. The cartilage should be gently crushed so that it is more malleable and less likely to be visible through the thinner skin overlying the radix. Two or more pieces of graft may be stacked and sutured together to increase height. The graft should be "fixed" into place to minimize postoperative malposition. This may be accomplished with a transcutaneous suture tied over a bolster and removed after 1 to 2 weeks. The suture is started through the skin just superior to the pocket for the graft and passed out through the access incision. It is passed through the graft outside the nose and then subcutaneously back up the dorsum and out of the skin just lateral to the other the end of the suture (Figure 18-2). A stiffer wire may also be placed through the skin and graft as alternate means of fixation. A simple dressing may suffice if tape is applied over the dorsal skin. The bolster an/or wire is frequently left in place for an average of 1 week to allow fixation of the graft but avoid a suture scar[1] (Figure 18-3).
- Radix augmentation at the superior portion of the nose will make the nose look shorter. In contrast, a low nasion that is augmented with a radix graft will increase nasal length.[2]
- *Pitfalls*:
  - Creation of too large a subcutaneous pocket for the graft without anchoring in place for a period of time by excessively wide dissection is likely to result in migration and ultimate malposition of the graft.
  - Radix augmentation may accentuate a narrow intercanthal distance, compromising facial aesthetics.
- *Tips*:
  - Dissection of the pocket should be limited and some means of holding the graft in place should be performed. Following ideal graft placement, the graft should be fixed in placed as indicated above.

REFERENCES

1. Becker D, Pastornek NJ. The radix graft in cosmetic rhinoplasty. *Arch Facial Plast Surg*. 2001;3:115.
2. Guyuron B. Dynamics in rhinoplasty. *Plast Reconstr Surg*. 2000;105:2257.

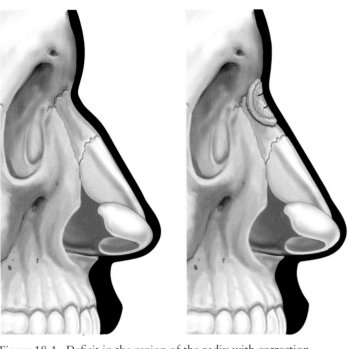

Figure 18-1. Deficit in the region of the radix with correction using a cartilage graft.

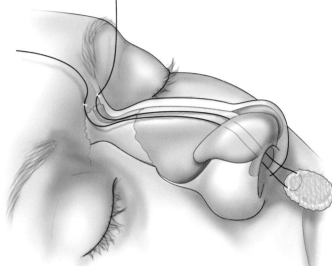

Figure 18-2. Placement of a radix graft using a bolstered suture.

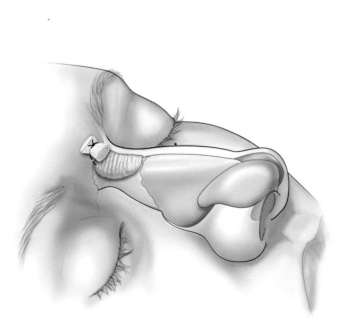

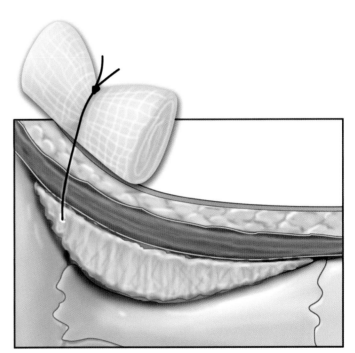

Figure 18-3. Bolster dressing used to hold the cartilage graft in place.

Chapter 19. Increasing Tip Projection

- *Indications*: Patients who lack nasal tip projection may be candidates for techniques that increase tip projection via the placement of sutures or grafts into the nasal tip structures (Figure 19-1). It should be noted that inadequate tip projection cannot be improved simply by reducing the dorsum. A true lateral photograph will better elucidate the need to increase tip projection.
- *Markings*: No specific skin markings need to be made preoperatively. However, a well-thought-out plan for surgery should be created including a tiered approach to achieve the desired result.
- *Approach*: The nasal tip may be approached via an endonasal or open nasal approach.

  - With the endonasal approach, bilateral intercartilaginous and infracartilaginous incisions are performed to allow the lower lateral cartilages to be freed from the skin of the overlying nasal tip. As two bipedicle flaps, they are then reflected outside the envelope of the nasal tip skin to be better visualized and manipulated. Sutures may be placed within each lower lateral cartilage or passed from one lower lateral cartilage to the other.
  - With the open nasal approach, a standard incision is made across the columella, extended up either side, and continued caudal to the inferior margins of the lower lateral cartilages. The nasal tip is dissected out as previously described.

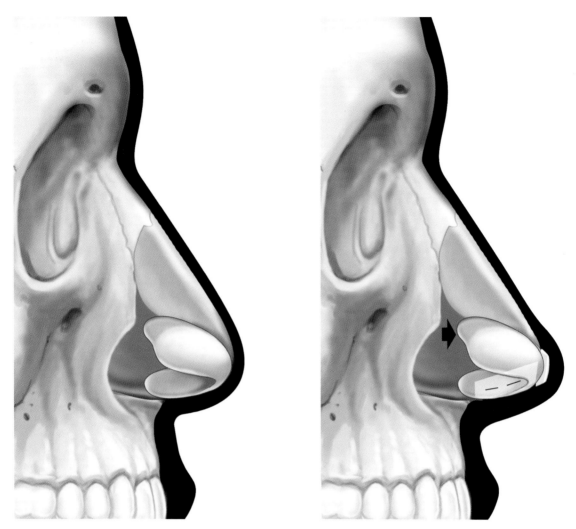

Figure 19-1. Underprojected nasal tip and its subsequent correction.

- *Techniques*: A graduated method of achieving increased tip projection is recommended and progresses from sutures to struts and grafts.[1,2]
  - *Tip sutures*: The simplest means of increasing tip projection is removal of any intervening interdomal tissue and suturing the middle crura to one another with medial crural sutures. Further projection can be achieved with interdomal or intradomal sutures. The lower lateral cartilage complex can also be elevated and sutured to either the septum or an anterior septal extension graft.
  - *Columellar strut*: If greater projection is desired, a cartilage strut may be placed into a pocket between the medial crura of the lower lateral cartilages to provide a supporting structure onto which the lower lateral cartilages may be reattached. An appropriate-sized pocket at the base of the columella is created to seat the cartilage graft, which is situated between the lateral footplates. The graft can be temporarily held in place with two 1½-in 25-gauge needles passed horizontally from lateral crus to graft to the opposite lateral crus (Figure 19-2). They are then sutured with 4-0 clear nylon or PDS sutures passed through all three structures and the knots buried between the graft and the lateral crus on one side of the columella. Two to three sutures should be used to prevent unwanted rotation of either the superior or inferior extent of the graft.
  - *Tip grafts*: To even further increase projection, an onlay graft can be sutured over the tip. If an endonasal approach is chosen, the graft may be placed through a marginal incision caudal to the inferior rim of the medial crura. Via an open approach, the graft should be sutured into place to minimize postoperative malposition. The graft material may be taken from any number of sources, including nasal septum, rib cage, or conchal bowl. It is shaped to the surgeon's wishes. Often, a pentagonal "shield" is created that sits in the midline just caudal to the true nasal tip (Figure 19-3). A more superiorly placed graft may also be used. For stiffer cartilage, the graft may be morcellized to soften it. The edges should also be beveled to minimize visibility beneath the skin. Simple sutures are placed at the corners of the graft to the underlying tip framework. Onlay grafts may be added to suturing techniques or columellar struts and several grafts may be placed overlapping one another or juxtaposed to one another to achieve the optimal tip projection and definition.
- *Postoperative management*: The nose is closed in the standard fashion with care taken not to disrupt the structure of the nasal tip. A dressing consisting of gradually longer Steri-strips placed across the dorsum from the radix to the supratip break and a single long Steri-strip placed down one sidewall, across the columella, and back up the other sidewall suffices as a dressing to hold the nasal tip in place. If a splint is desired in concert with the tapes, it may be custom contoured and added on top.
- *Pitfalls*:
  - If a columellar strut is placed to the level of the anterior nasal spine, it may remain loose and create a clicking sensation as it moves across the anterior nasal spine. This can be avoided by using a floating strut that stops short of the spine or by securing the graft against the spine.
  - The skin in an open approach should be temporarily sutured while tip projection is assessed. If the tip is assessed with the skin pulled over the cartilage, but not completely closed, the surgeon will be disappointed by the loss of projection that occurs with complete skin closure.
- *Tips*:
  - Exposure of the lower lateral cartilages may be achieved via either an endonasal or open nasal approach. However, successful modification of the complex nasal tip may be better achieved via the open approach.
  - Avoiding violation of the underlying nasal mucosa when placing intradomal sutures within the middle crura may be difficult. Sutures may be more easily placed by flattening the arc of the middle crura with a finger before placing the suture.
  - To minimize displacement of a columellar strut, the pocket for the strut should not extend down to the anterior nasal spine unless a large amount of tip projection is required. In these cases, an intraoral buccal mucosal approach gives access to secure the base of the graft to the anterior nasal spine.
  - It is useful to save the fascial tissue removed from the tip cartilages. It can be useful to cover tip grafts and reduce the likelihood of graft visibility.

REFERENCES

1. Rohrich RJ, Muzaffar AR. Primary rhinoplasty. In: Achauer BM, Eriksson E, Vander Kolk C, et al., eds. *Plastic Surgery: Indications, Operations, and Outcomes*. Volume 5. St. Louis, MO: Mosby; 2000:2631–2672.
2. Tebbets JB. Shaping and positioning of the nasal tip without surgical disruption: A systematic approach. *Plast Reconstr Surg.* 1994;94(1):61–77.

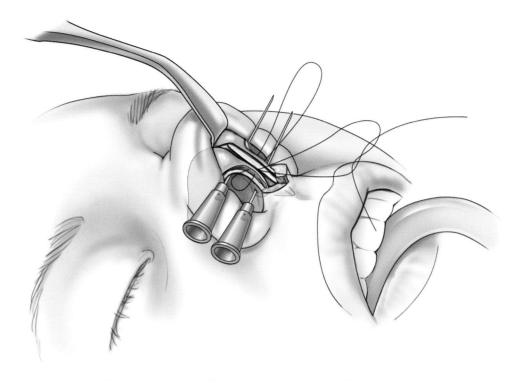

Figure 19-2. Temporary fixation of a columella strut with 25-gauge needles while sutures are placed.

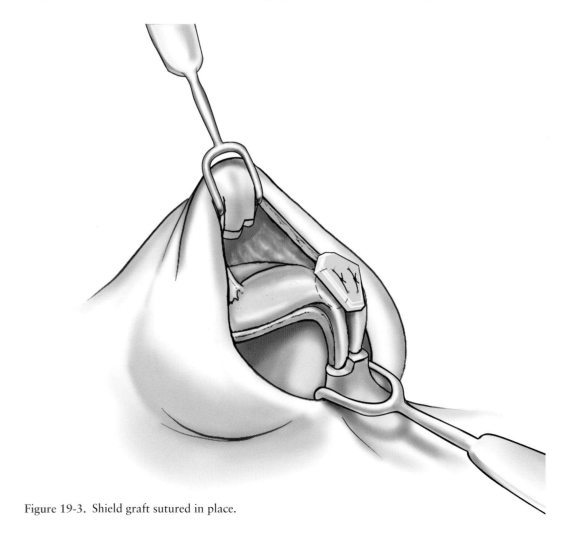

Figure 19-3. Shield graft sutured in place.

Chapter 20. Decreasing Tip Projection

- *Indications*: Patients with increased projection of the nasal tip may be candidates for a number of specific interventions to decrease tip projection and improve facial balance (Figure 20-1). This is often not easy to achieve and a careful preoperative determination of the patient's problem should be made. Specific factors that may contribute to the increased projection include the length of either the medial or lateral crura of the lower lateral cartilages, distance from the footplates of the medial crura to the anterior nasal spine, connections between the medial crura and the caudal septum, and connections between the lateral crura and the caudal border of the upper lateral cartilages.

- *Markings*: No specific markings need to be made preoperatively. However, a well-thought-out plan for surgery should be created.

- *Approach*: Maneuvers to decrease projection of the tip are best addressed with an open approach. Via an endonasal approach, the hemi- or full transfixion incision will disrupt the connections between the medial crura and the caudal septum. Continuing the mucosal incision laterally as an intercartilaginous incision will further disjoin the lateral crura from the caudal margin of the upper lateral cartilages. For the open approach, a standard incision is made across the waist of the columellar skin and extended into bilateral rim incisions for optimal exposure of the components of the nasal tip.

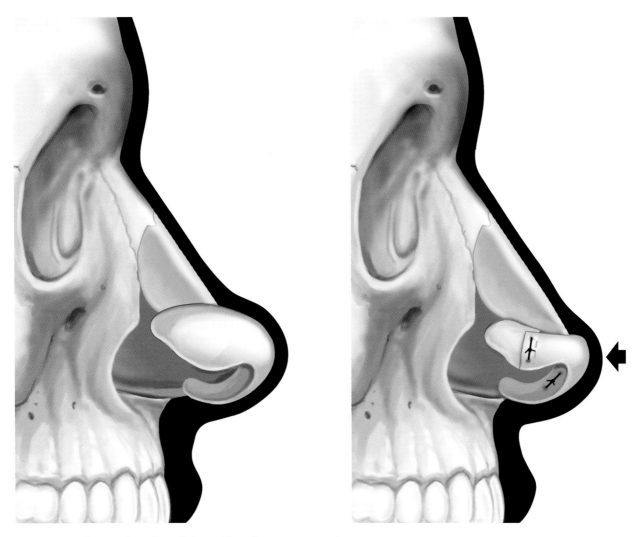

Figure 20-1. Overprojected nasal tip and its subsequent correction.

- *Techniques*: To decrease tip projection, it is important to address the anatomic structures that contribute to support of the nasal tip. These include the skin over the lower lateral cartilages, the position of the lower lateral cartilages themselves, the fibrous attachments between the lower and upper lateral cartilages, and those between the lower lateral cartilages and the caudal septum. A graduated method of decreasing tip projection is recommended as described below.[1,2]
  - *Medial/middle crural release*: For minimal deformity, release of ligaments and placement of sutures between the middle crura and caudal septum will set back the lower lateral cartilage complex to a certain degree. If further retrusion is necessary, alternate maneuvers will be required.
  - *Cephalic trim*: Excision of a portion of the cephalic margin of the lower lateral cartilage will further disrupt support of the nasal tip (Figure 20-2). Following detachment of the tip from the more superior structures, projection is left to the length and strength of the lateral cartilages. A medial crural-septal suture may be used to secure the tip in a more posterior position (Figure 20-3).
  - *Septal extension graft (see Chapter 23)*: A septal extension graft can be used as a stabilizing structure to which the tip can be sutured to reinforce the desired degree of projection.
  - *Crural transection*: Shortening of the lateral arms of the lower lateral cartilages will reduce the projection of these elements of the nasal tip. This is accomplished by freeing the cartilage from the skin and nasal mucosa, transecting and overlapping the lower lateral cartilage, and resuturing the ends in their overlapped position (Figure 20-4). Cartilage transection to decrease tip projection may be done at the level of either the medial or lateral crura. The lateral crura are frequently addressed before the medial crura because they provide a greater contribution to tip support in many patients. Loss of tip projection may increase alar flaring, and this is addressed after the tip is in its final position. If alar flaring is present, an alar resection may be necessary.
- *Postoperative management*: A single Steri-strip placed down one sidewall, across the columella, and back up the other sidewall suffices as a dressing to hold the repositioned columella in place.
- *Pitfalls*:
  - Deprojection of the nasal tip may make the dorsum appear too high requiring dorsal reduction.[3]
  - Alar retraction may occur following trim of the cephalic border of the lower lateral cartilages.
  - Alar flaring may result from decreasing tip projection. If this occurs, it should be addressed at surgery.
- *Tips*:
  - A careful preoperative examination should attempt to identify the anatomic structure(s) most responsible for the increased tip projection.
  - If alar retraction is noted following trim of the cephalic margins of the lower lateral cartilages, the excised piece of cartilage may be preserved and used to bolster the remaining lower lateral cartilage. A pocket is dissected beneath the upper border and the excised piece sutured back under the remaining portion with interrupted 5-0 PDS suture. This serves to stiffen the support of the alar rim and blend with the upper lateral cartilage.

REFERENCES

1. Rohrich RJ, Muzaffar AR. Primary rhinoplasty. In: Achauer BM, Eriksson E, Vander Kolk C, et al., eds. *Plastic Surgery: Indications, Operations, and Outcomes.* Volume 5. St. Louis, MO: Mosby; 2000:2631–2672.
2. Tebbets JB. Shaping and positioning of the nasal tip without surgical disruption: A systematic approach. *Plast Reconstr Surg.* 1994;94(1):61–77.
3. Guyuron B. Dynamic interplays during rhinoplasty. *Clin Plast Surg.* 1996;23:223–231.

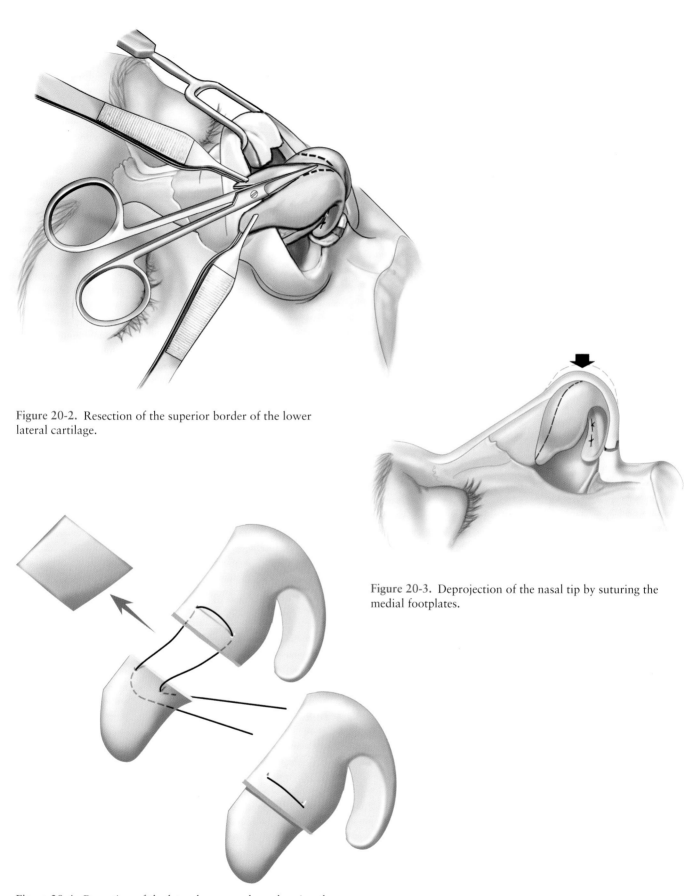

Figure 20-2. Resection of the superior border of the lower lateral cartilage.

Figure 20-3. Deprojection of the nasal tip by suturing the medial footplates.

Figure 20-4. Resection of the lateral crura and overlapping the transected ends.

Chapter 21. Increasing Tip Rotation

- *Indications*: Patients in whom there is little or no nostril show likely have excessive downward rotation of either the nose itself or the nasal tip (Figure 21-1). The amount of rotation is best described by the angle between the nose and upper lip. The normal value for the nasolabial angle in females is approximately 100 degrees to 105 degrees and in males it is approximately 95 degrees to 100 degrees. Patients in whom this angle is too acute may be candidates for techniques that rotate the tip upwards. The position of the nose is determined by the elements that stabilize the nasal tip. These include the skin over the lower lateral cartilages, the position of the lower lateral cartilages themselves, the fibrous attachments between the lower and upper lateral cartilages, and those between the lower lateral cartilages and the caudal septum. Lateral crura that are positioned more obliquely within the nasal tip and alar margin contribute to decreased tip rotation. Hyperactivity of the *depressor septi nasi* muscle can also be an important factor contributing to decreased rotation of the nasal tip, especially during smiling. An "overactive" depressor septi muscle that contributes to drooping of the nasal tip is diagnosed by the "smile test" (ie, the nasal tip drops slightly when the patient smiles). Division of this muscle has been described as a treatment for the patient with a positive smile test.[1]

- *Markings*: No specific markings need to be made preoperatively. A well-thought-out plan for surgery should be created. The estimated degree of change in the nasolabial angle is helpful in predicting the maneuvers that will be required to effect this change.

- *Approach*: The major contributors to the nasocolumellar angle are the caudal end of the septum and the anterior nasal spine of the maxilla. Rarely are the middle crura of the lower lateral cartilage a significant factor. Both of these structures can be approached through either a closed or an open approach. With an open approach, the skin is undermined to free the lower lateral cartilages of restrictive forces. The individual lower lateral cartilage complexes can be separated by dissecting through the loose soft tissue between them to allow visualization of the caudal septum. The anterior spine is found by dissecting inferiorly to the maxillary bone. With a closed approach, a hemi- or complete transection incision allows similar exposure of these structures.

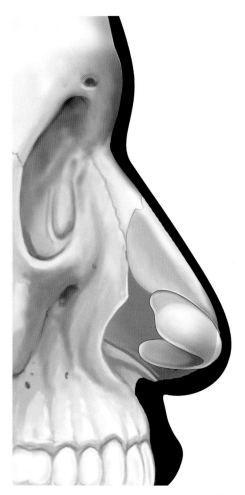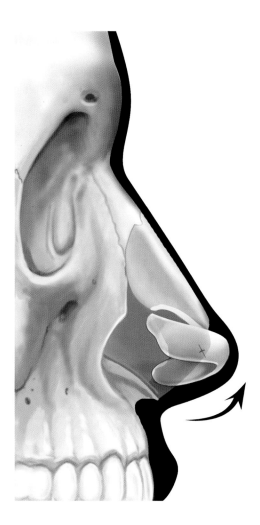

Figure 21-1. Under-rotated nasal tip and its correction.

- *Technique*: Small increases in tip rotation may be achieved by simple excision of the cephalic border of the lower lateral cartilages (Figure 21-2). Trimming a portion of the cephalic border of the lateral crura of the lower lateral cartilages is performed as a means of reducing the fibrous attachments between the lateral crura and upper lateral cartilages. In addition, the space created by the excision allows the more inferior portions of the cartilage to rotate in a counterclockwise direction to fill the space. Calipers are used to measure the amount of cartilage from the cephalic aspect of the lower lateral cartilage that is to be left behind to maintain support of the external nasal valve. In general, no less than 4 mm to 6 mm should be left for support. A #15 blade is used to incise the cartilage along its length being careful to avoid injury to the underlying nasal mucosa. The portion to be resected is then grasped with forceps from either end and removed with either the scalpel or a fine scissors. It should be kept on the operative field in moist saline gauze in case it is required as an onlay graft.
  - The lower lateral cartilages may also be rotated superiorly by the use of sutures placed between the medial crura and the septum to fix the lower lateral cartilages in a more cephalad position (Figure 21-3). This suture engages the nasal tip and is attached to the anterocaudal septum. As it is tightened, it rotates the tip in a counterclockwise direction. The knot is set at the desired angle of tip rotation.
  - Another means of rotating the nasal tip is by transection of the lateral crural complex. The skin over the lateral aspect of the lateral crura may be undermined and the attachments of the lower lateral cartilage to the accessory cartilages transected in a vertical direction. To maintain or increase the amount of rotation of the nasal tip, a columellar strut graft may be needed. The graft should be taken from a source that provides straighter, denser cartilage (septum, rib) rather the ear, which is more contoured and malleable. The graft material is placed between the medial crura of the lower lateral cartilages and sutured to both to provide intrinsic support. A septal extension graft can also be used to control the tip rotation. This should be a straight, large, rigid piece of cartilage that will be able to be secured to the septum and the medial and middle crura. The septal end can be secured with PDS sutures, and then the tip rotation is set and secured by suturing the septal extension graft to the middle crura. This graft maintains the desired projection. Septal cartilage is ideal because it is strong and straight. Rib cartilage may warp, and ear cartilage is too soft. A 0.5-mm PDS foil may be used to add rigidity to the ear cartilage or minimize warping on rib cartilage.

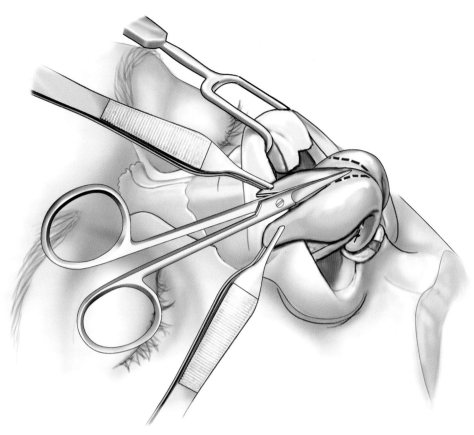

Figure 21-2. Cephalic trim of the lower lateral cartilages.

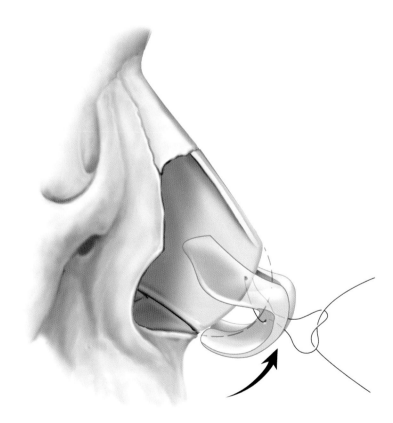

Figure 21-3. Tip rotation using caudal septal suture.

- Either a prominent or weak caudal septum will affect tip rotation. Several millimeters of caudal septum may be resected to produce changes in tip projection (Figure 21-4). If this is performed more anteriorly, some increased rotation of the tip will be anticipated. If performed more posteriorly, close to the anterior nasal spine, a greater deepening of the infranasal region will be achieved resulting in a more acute nasolabial angle.
- A weak nasal spine that produces an acute nasolabial angle can be enhanced with a graft of cartilage placed between the lower lateral cartilages, which extend caudal to the medial crura of the lower lateral cartilage. This graft may stop just short of the anterior nasal spine or may be sutured to it to further prevent migration. Some surgeons elect to augment the maxilla along the inferior aspect of the piriform aperture with either a rolled piece of autogenous fascia or alloplast (ProPlast or GoreTex). This technique generally warrants an approach via an upper gingivobuccal sulcus incision.
- Finally, one or more of the depressor septi nasi fascicles may be detached from their origin on the anterior nasal spine and insertion on the septum (Figure 21-5). This may be accomplished through an intranasal approach, in which the muscle fibers may be taken off the medial crus footplate and septal cartilage. Additionally, separation of the muscle fibers off the anterior nasal spine may be accomplished through either the existing intranasal approach or through a separate gingivobuccal sulcus incision.
- *Postoperative management*: A single Steri-strip placed down one sidewall, across the columella, and back up the other sidewall suffices as a dressing to hold the repositioned tip-columella complex in place.
- *Pitfalls*:
  - Rotation of the nasal tip should always be considered carefully. As the tip rotates cephalad, the length of the dorsum shortens and the amount of nostril show increases.
  - Resection of the cephalic portion of the lateral crura of the lower lateral cartilages disrupts the fibrous attachments to the upper lateral cartilages and may weaken tip support.
  - Resection of the caudal septum may rotate the nasal tip upwards. This may be a desired change, but should certainly be anticipated in the event it is not.
  - Any tissue placed along the piriform aperture may become visible when the patient smiles or may restrict animation of the face.
  - Alloplast may migrate or become exposed, warranting removal and ultimate replacement if still desired.
- *Tips*:
  - When performing cephalic resection from the lower lateral cartilages, it is important to measure from the inferior aspect of the cartilage and leave at least 4 mm to 6 mm of remaining cartilage. It is important that what remains is symmetric, not what is removed.
  - If indicated, resection of the caudal septum should be performed before harvesting septum to avoid leaving the caudal strut of septum narrower than the recommended 1 cm.
  - In addition to augmentation of the caudal septum with a graft, separate pieces of cartilage may be placed beneath the skin of the columella to achieve further correction as necessary.
  - Alloplastic augmentation should be avoided if possible since safe, reliable alternatives exist.

REFERENCE

1. Rohrich RJ, Huynh B, Muzzaffar AR, et al. Importance of the depressor septi nasi muscle in rhinoplasty: Anatomic study and clinical application. *Plast Reconstr Surg.* 2000;105:376.

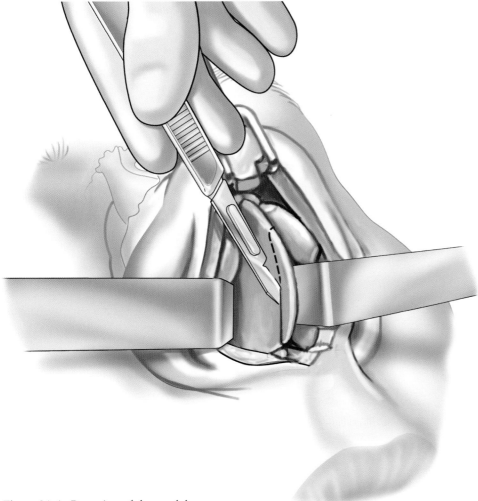

Figure 21-4. Resection of the caudal septum.

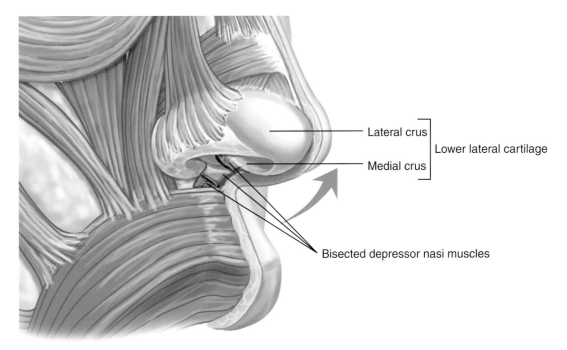

Lateral crus

Medial crus

Lower lateral cartilage

Bisected depressor nasi muscles

Figure 21-5. Transection of the depressor nasi muscles.

Chapter 22. Decreasing Tip Rotation

- *Indications*: Patients with increased upwards rotation of the nose present with a short nose and an excessive amount of nostril show (Figure 22-1). Fortunately, this is not one of the more commonly encountered problems. Analysis of the face involves lateral inspection of the nasolabial angle. As stated earlier, the normal nasolabial angle for women is approximately 100 degrees to 105 degrees and that for men is 95 degrees to 100 degrees. Another important measurement is the nasofacial angle, which lies between the dorsal nasal line and the facial plane. Here, the values are roughly 36 degrees for males and 34 degrees for females.

- *Markings*: No specific markings need to be made preoperatively. However, a well-thought-out plan for surgery should be created. A closed or open approach may be favored for counterclockwise rotation of the nose.

- *Approach*:
  - As with the under-rotated nose, the skin over the lower lateral cartilages must be undermined to free the cartilage from forces that serve to restrict desired movement.
  - Conservative resection of the cephalic portion of the lower lateral cartilage serves to address the excess volume commonly seen in these patients. By performing a full transfixion incision with the closed approach, the two major contributors to the nasolabial angle can be addressed, namely the caudal septum and the anterior nasal spine. Rarely are the middle crura of the lower lateral cartilage a significant contributing factor.

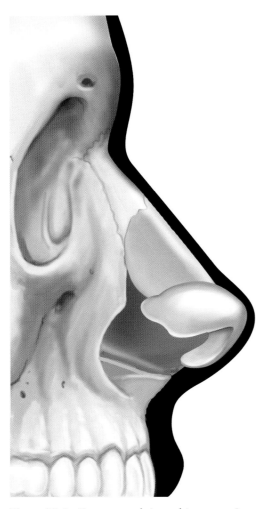
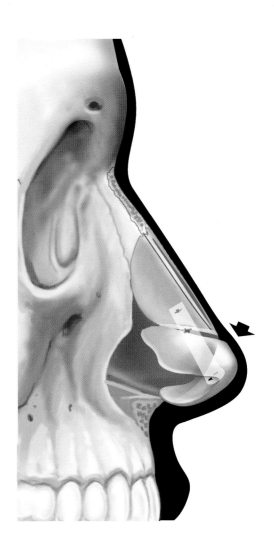

Figure 22-1. Over-rotated tip and its correction.

- The lower lateral cartilages are freed of their attachments to (1) the upper lateral cartilages with a limited cephalic trim, (2) the caudal septum by performing a transfixion incision, and (3) the piriform aperture via a vertical incision in the region of the sesamoid cartilages. A septal extension graft of cartilage harvested from either the septum or the rib and fixed to both the dorsal septum and medial crura will serve to push the tip inferiorly and derotate the nose (Figure 22-2). Septal cartilage is ideal as ear cartilage is often not strong enough and costal cartilage tends to warp. A 0.5-mm PDS foil may help reinforce weak cartilage and reduce warping.
- Separation of the lower lateral cartilages from each other in the midline and dissecting the intervening loose tissue will enable visualization of the caudal septum. To make room for the rotated medial crura of the lower lateral cartilages, the posterior aspect of the caudal septum may also need to be resected. This will also decrease the nasolabial angle.
- Proceeding inferiorly to the maxilla will identify the anterior nasal spine. With a closed approach, a hemi- or complete transection incision allows similar exposure of these structures. Alternatively, a limited, midline gingivobuccal incision can be used. A prominent nasal spine that produces an obtuse nasolabial angle can be de-emphasized by shortening its length or deepening its anterior surface with a rongeur (Figure 22-3).
- Additionally, one or more sutures from the caudal septum may be passed to more anterior points on the lower lateral cartilages to direct these structures more posteriorly.

- *Postoperative management*: A single strip of tape placed down one sidewall, across the columella, and back up the other sidewall suffices as a dressing to hold the repositioned columella in place.
- *Pitfalls*:
  - Clockwise rotation of the nasal tip may cause the nostrils to flare outward. If warranted, this can be corrected with limited bilateral resection of the alar base.
  - The dorsum will need to be evaluated after clockwise rotation because it may require reduction to maintain aesthetic balance.
- *Tips*:
  - Incremental progression will guide the amount of rotation needed to maximize the aesthetic result.[1,2]
  - As the nasal tip rotates inferiorly, the dorsum may become more prominent and may need to be reduced as described earlier.

REFERENCES

1. Rohrich RJ, Muzaffar AR. Primary rhinoplasty. In: Achauer BM, Eriksson E, Vander Kolk C, et al., eds. *Plastic Surgery: Indications, Operations, and Outcomes.* Volume 5. St. Louis, MO: Mosby; 2000:2631–2672.
2. Tebbets JB. Shaping and positioning of the nasal tip without surgical disruption: A systematic approach. *Plast Reconstr Surg.* 1994;94(1):61–77.

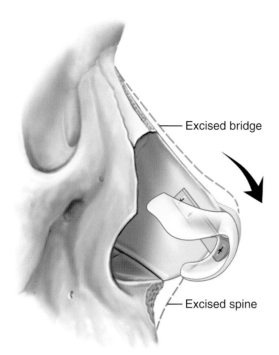

Figure 22-2. Clockwise rotation of the nasal tip by excision and graft placement.

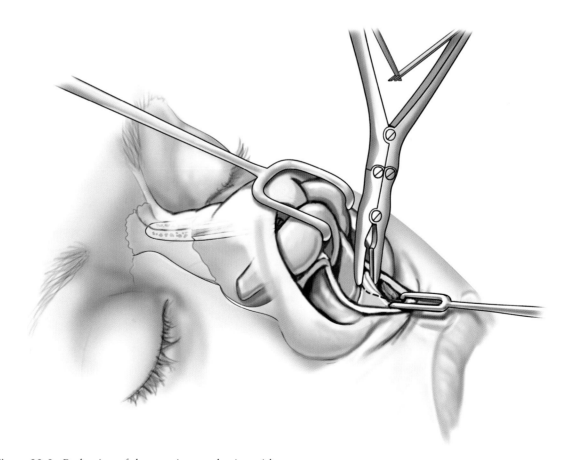

Figure 22-3. Reduction of the anterior nasal spine with a rongeur.

Chapter 23. Upper Lateral Cartilages: Grafting Techniques

- The cartilaginous portion of the dorsum contains the transition zone between the upper lateral cartilages and the midline septum. On cross section, this is not a sharp angle but a well-supported and gradual curve. With resection of the dorsal septum, collapse of the middle vault may occur as the upper lateral cartilages fall towards the septum in a more acute manner. In the absence of structurally sound upper lateral cartilages, collapse of the nasal sidewall or asymmetry can occur and require reconstruction with a cartilage graft of similar quality. Spreader grafts are indicated to reconstruct compromised dorsal aesthetic lines, open roof deformities, and nasal deviations.[1]

- *Assessment and Markings*: No specific markings are necessary for planning and placement of cartilage grafts for support of the middle cartilaginous vault. The presence of a nasal deviation, open roof deformity, or compromised dorsal aesthetic outline should be identified. The grafts will ultimately lie on either side of the dorsal septum. If upper lateral cartilage collapse has caused a loss of a dorsal aesthetic line, the septal graft can be placed more dorsal on the septum to restore this lost fullness. Spreader grafts can also be fashioned to extend beyond the anterior septal angle as a septal extension graft. In this case the extension graft serves as a stable strut to which the lower lateral cartilage (tip) complex can be sutured to control nasal tip rotation and projection. Septal cartilage is the ideal material for spreader grafts; however, rib or ear cartilage can be used if septal cartilage is unavailable. The inherent warping nature of the rib cartilage may be advantageous in correcting nasal deviation.[2]

- *Approach*: Approaching the upper lateral cartilages may be achieved via either a closed or an open rhinoplasty. With an open approach, a transcolumellar incision is continued superiorly and laterally along the infracartilaginous alar rim. Dissection above the lower lateral cartilages and along the midline dorsum may be extended laterally to identify the upper lateral cartilages. A clear junction between the midline septum and upper lateral cartilages is often difficult to appreciate. If the caudal septum is approached by separating the lower lateral cartilages and dissecting along the septum in a submucosal plane, the upper lateral cartilages may be identified by reflecting the mucosa closest to the dorsum.

- *Technique*: Cartilage sufficient for structural support is harvested from the septum if it is present. This should be determined in the preoperative consult. Costal cartilage may also be used for this purpose and is favored by some. Conchal cartilage is frequently more convoluted, thinner, and softer making it less ideal for spreader grafts. However, with the introduction of the PDS flexible plate (Mentor™) as a reinforcing material, its use may be expanded in this indication.

  ○ Septal cartilage may be harvested through a separate unilateral mucosal incision leaving the most dorsal portion of the septum untouched for later positioning of the grafts. The caudal portion of the septum is then transected preserving the contralateral mucosa to minimize the risk of a perforation. Dissection is continued posteriorly and inferiorly on both sides of the septum. A strut of at least 1 cm is preserved to maintain support to the lower half of the nose (Figure 23-1). Septal cartilage may also be harvested via a caudal approach between the medial crura of the lower lateral cartilages (Figure 23-2).

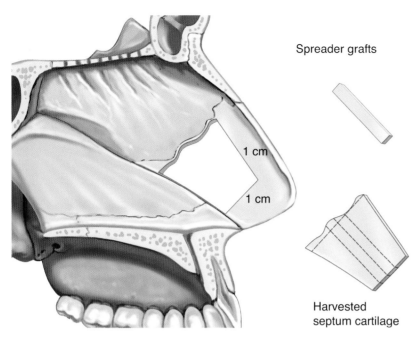

Spreader grafts

1 cm

1 cm

Harvested
septum cartilage

Figure 23-1 Harvested nasal septum for use as spreader grafts.

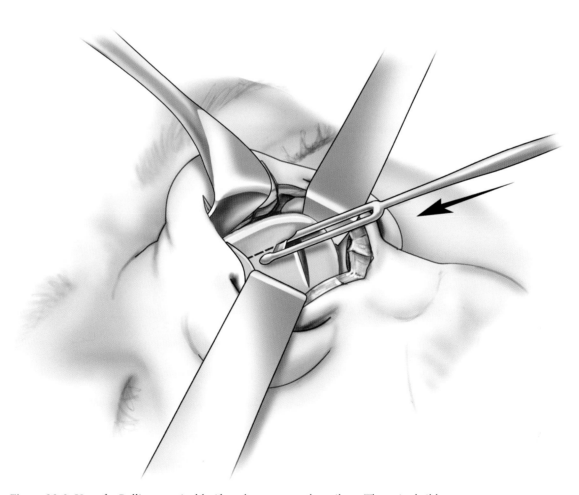

Figure 23-2 Use of a Ballinger swivel knife to harvest septal cartilage. The paired ribbon retractors protect the mucosa.

○ Costal cartilage is harvested from the more medial portions of the ribcage as described earlier.

○ Conchal cartilage can be reinforced with a PDS flexible plate to add rigidity and eliminate curvature expanding its application as a spreader or extension graft.

○ Following harvest of sufficient graft material, one or two absorbable 4-0 gut mattress sutures should be placed across the mucosal septum. If the mucosa is not approximated there is a potential space for blood and fluid accumulation.

○ For spreader grafts, the harvested cartilage is placed onto a sterile cutting surface so that two equal grafts may be fabricated. This is best done with a fresh #15 scalpel blade. The size of the grafts should measure 20 mm to 25 mm in length and 3 mm to 4 mm in height and width.

○ The spreader grafts are positioned on either side of the dorsal septum medial to the upper lateral cartilages (Figure 23-3). The superior end of each graft should lie beneath the caudal end of the bony vault (Figure 23-4). With the closed technique, two tunnels are created along each side of the most dorsal aspect of the septum. If a tight pocket is created, it is conceivable that sutures may not need to be placed. With the open technique, two or three sutures will serve to hold the grafts in place. Since both suture needles should pass through five layers (right upper lateral cartilage, right spreader graft, septum, left spreader graft, and left upper lateral cartilage), it is helpful to set up the construct using two 25-gauge needles passed across all components of the dorsal septum—one cranial and one caudal (Figure 23-5). Alternatively, each spreader graft can be sutured independently with approximation of the upper lateral cartilages performed after placement of the spreader grafts. The grafts are sutured into place with two or three clear, 5-0 permanent monofilament or PDS sutures. One suture will generally not suffice since it allows the grafts to rotate within the sagittal plane. The knots may be buried between one of the layers to minimize their palpability. Before completion, the reconstructed dorsum should be checked to confirm that it is smooth and that none of the graft edges are palpable beneath the dorsal nasal skin envelope.

○ Autospreader grafts can be used when a significant amount of cartilaginous septum is reduced and excess upper lateral cartilage remains above the leading edge of the septum. This redundant cartilage is folded medially towards the septum and sutured together.[3] In this instance, the upper lateral cartilages serve as their own spreader grafts to increase the internal valve angle.

○ Onlay graft material that is used to camouflage deficient upper lateral cartilage should be morcellized or beveled at its edges to minimize the risk of visibility. It may be sutured at its medial aspect to avoid postoperative migration.

• *Postoperative management*: An internal nasal splint composed of either resorbable or nonresorbable material should be used postoperatively. Resorbable material includes Gelfoam sponge; nonresorbable material includes plain petroleum gauze or petroleum gauze with bismuth (Xeroform®). Antibiotics should be used in patients with nonresorbable packing to minimize the risk of infection and toxic shock syndrome.

• *Pitfalls*:

○ Preservation of the nasal mucosa is important and care should be exercised in dissecting the upper lateral cartilages and nasal septum. This may be done with a Freer or Cottle elevator being careful to maintain contact between the tip of the instrument and the cartilage.

○ Over-resection of the upper lateral cartilages, in an attempt to lower the cartilaginous nasal dorsum, will further weaken the support of the middle vault.

• *Tips*:

○ Small, incremental changes in the upper lateral cartilages should be performed to avoid over-resection.

○ Once the spreader grafts are positioned along the septum and held in place with two 25-gauge needles, it is helpful to suture the caudal end first since it easier to visualize.

○ If the graft(s) are well sutured into place, it is usually safe to save lateral osteotomies and fracturing to the end especially if the osteotomies are complete and the force needed to move the nasal bones is minor.

REFERENCES

1. Sheen JH. Spreader graft: A method of reconstructing the roof of the middle nasal vault following rhinoplasty. *Plast Reconstr Surg.* 1984;73:230.

2. Byrd HS, Andochick S, Copit S. Septal extension grafts: A method for controlling tip projection and shape. *Plast Reconstr Surg.* 1997;100:999.

3. Seyhan A. Method for middle vault reconstruction in primary rhinoplasty: Upper lateral cartilage bending. *Plast Reconstr Surg.* 1997;100:1941–1943.

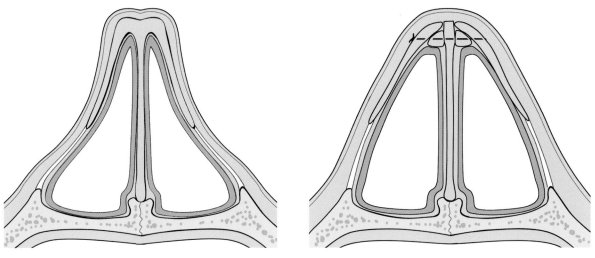

Figure 23-3. Placement and function of spreader grafts.

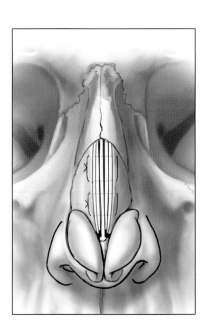

Figure 23-4. Dorsal septum with spreader grafts in place.

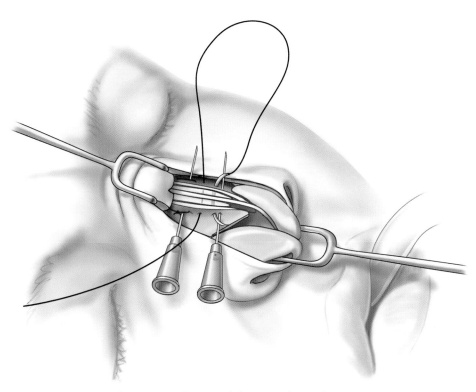

Figure 23-5. Use of syringe needles to stabilize spreader grafts.

Chapter 24. The Wide Tip: Suture Techniques

- *Indications*: In contrast to excision, techniques for suturing cartilage have the advantage of being nondestructive and reversible. Patients in whom the lower lateral cartilages are deformed or malpositioned require reconstruction, which in some part relies on sutures placed either within the domes of the cartilages, between the domes of the middle crura, and/or from the cartilages to surrounding structures. Sutures are frequently used to alter the curvature or position of the cartilage (Figure 24-1). Common maneuvers address domes that are too wide or domes that are situated too far from each other. Patients in whom these maneuvers are particular useful are those with wide or boxy tips. Similar techniques may be used for lateral deflections of the septum.

- *Markings*: Preoperatively, the position of all three components of the lower lateral cartilages should be identified beneath the skin envelope. The medial crura extend predominantly up the length of the columella. They may or may not contribute to excessive show of the columella on lateral view. The middle crura are perhaps the most visible and form the tip-defining points on frontal view. The lateral crura may extend along the alar rims and rotate superiorly.

- *Approach*: Access to the lower lateral cartilages may be achieved via an open or closed approach to the nasal tip. However, many surgeons believe that better exposure is afforded by the open approach. Recent reports have outlined combined approaches that spare the patient a transcolumellar incision but allow adequate visualization of the nasal tip.[1] The anatomy of the lower lateral cartilages should be carefully assessed to determine if the pathology is due primarily to a widened dome arc, increased divergence between the two domes, or a combination of the two.[2,3]

- *Technique*: The choice of suture for tip modification is a personal one. The material should pass easily through the cartilage causing the least trauma and last long enough to prevent relapse. Either a permanent, monofilament suture, such clear nylon, or a long-acting dissolvable suture, such as polydioxanone (PDS) may be used. Shorter acting sutures, such as plain gut, and braided sutures, such as polyglactin (Vicryl®), are not recommended.

- *Tip narrowing sutures*:
  - A medial footplate suture is a mattress suture that approximates the medial crura. Intervening soft tissue is usually dissected prior to suture placement to maximize the degree of columellar narrowing and minimize the inferior protrusion of the columella (columellar hang).
  - A medial crura-septal suture is used to increase or decrease nasal tip projection and rotation. The medial crura are isolated and a suture is passed through the medial crura and the caudal septum to secure the tip in its desired position. If the sutures are placed through the posterior crura and moved anteriorly, tip projection increases and cephalic (counterclockwise) tip rotation occurs. If the anterior medial crura are secured posterior to the caudal septum, tip projection decreases and tip rotation moves in a caudal (clockwise) direction.
  - A middle crural suture is similar to the medial crural suture but is placed more anterior, near the tip. This serves to provide more tip narrowing and support than the medial crural suture.
  - An intradomal suture spans the domal arch anterior to the vestibular lining (Figure 24-2). A clear, monofilament suture is placed in a mattress pattern with the knots kept medially where they are less likely to be palpable. The entrance and exit points should be spaced appropriately. Points that are too close together will not impart sufficient folding of the crura, while those that gather too much intervening cartilage will create too severe a deformation. Care should be taken that the suture does not catch the underlying vestibular mucosa.

Pre-operative

Post-operative

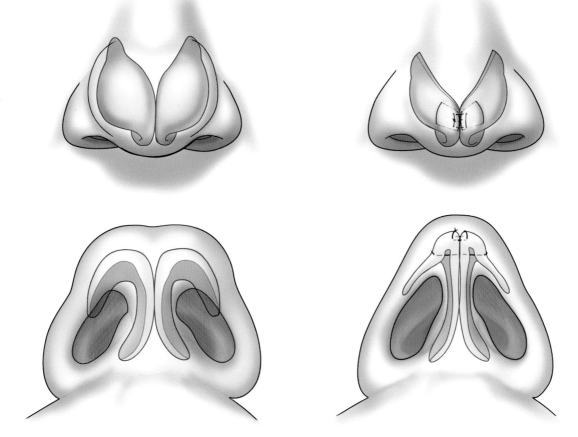

Figure 24-1. Boxy nasal tip and correction using interdomal suture and cephalic trim.

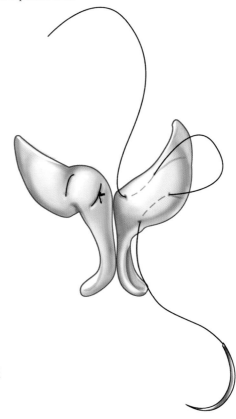

Figure 24-2. Horizontal mattress intradomal suture used to narrow the middle crura.

The effects of this suture are tip narrowing, increased lobular size, increased tip projection, and interdomal narrowing. The lateral crural concavity that occurs with this suture may be noted and an alar rim graft may be needed to avoid alar retraction or compromise of the external nasal valve. The exact location of the interdomal suture will affect the crura so placement is important. More cephalic placement results in slight upward rotation of lateral crura. Mid-domal placement narrows the domes without rotation, while caudal placement results in slight downward crural displacement. This suture is indicated when the interdomal distance is ideal but the domal arches are too wide.

○ An interdomal suture is a horizontal mattress suture between the domes that approximates the most anterior point of each crura. This suture will narrow the tip and increase length (Figure 24-3). This suture is more effective at approximating the domes than the intradomal suture. As with the intradomal suture, the exact location of the interdomal suture will affect the crura so placement is important. Cephalic placement will result in slight again upward rotation of the lateral crura. Mid-domal placement will narrow the domes without rotation, and caudal placement results in slight downward crural displacement. This suture is used when the domal arches are optimally shaped but are too far apart. The suture can be used alone or in combination with the intradomal suture.

○ A lateral crural suture is placed as a horizontal mattress suture that spans from the cephalic portion of one lateral crus through the caudal septum to the opposite lateral crus and is tied over the septum at the desired tension. The purpose of this suture is to narrow the lateral crura and elongate the nose.

○ A lateral crural spanning suture is a horizontal mattress suture that extends over convex portions of the lateral crura (Figure 24-4). The suture at the ends of the mattress pattern should be spaced 3 mm to 4 mm apart to support adequate tension across the suture. As it is tightened, the underlying lateral crural convexity is flattened or even made concave, if desired. Scoring the cartilage on the side opposite the desired change will facilitate the deformation. This suture will also result in increased tip projection.[4]

○ *Suture sequence*: The sequence of suture placement stabilizes the central nose first with placement of medial and middle crural sutures as indicated. These sutures stabilize the base of the tip. Domal sutures are then placed followed by lateral crural sutures if necessary. The medial crural septal suture is then placed to set the nasal projection followed by the tip-rotation suture.

○ *Tip-dorsum relationship*: In general, the domes of the lower lateral cartilages should project 6 mm to 8 mm above the level of the dorsal septum.

• *Postoperative management*: A standard dressing of Steri-strips along the dorsum and around the tip is recommended as a postoperative dressing.

• *Pitfalls*:
  ○ Definition in the tip is difficult to achieve in the patient with thick, glabrous skin. In contrast, care should be exercised in the patient with thin skin for fear of necrosis from skin flaps that are too thin.
  ○ Following the placement of sutures to narrow the nasal tip, the alar rims should be inspected to make sure they are not elevated as a side effect.
  ○ Placement of an intradomal suture can deflect the lateral crura too far medially, causing collapse of the external nasal valve. The problem can be corrected by supporting the lateral crura with an alar batten graft.
  ○ For all sutures, care should be taken not to over-perforate the cartilage with excessive passes of the suture and not to damage the cartilage with excessive traction.
  ○ For interdomal sutures, a tip that is too pointed can occur if the domes are brought too close together.
  ○ For lateral crura sutures, excessive flattening or curvature can result if the suture is tied too tight.
  ○ For crural-septal sutures, either over- or under-rotation or over- or under-projection can occur if the suture is not placed in an ideal location.

• *Tips*:
  ○ Tip reconstruction should be chosen for the proper patient. Any unintended effects of suture placement should be considered in addition to the intended ones.
  ○ For transcrural sutures, excessive narrowing should be considered and avoided.
  ○ Alar rim grafts should be inserted when numerous tip-suturing methods are employed since the external valves become weak and the ala may appear concave and retracted.
  ○ When placing mattress sutures over convex lateral crura, it is helpful to flatten the cartilage with one's finger to reduce the chance of the suture perforating the vestibular mucosa.

REFERENCES

1. Bravo FG, Schwarze HP. Closed-open rhinoplasty with extended lip dissection: A new concept and classification of rhinoplasty. *Plast Reconstr Surg.* 2008 Sep;122: 944–950.
2. Weber S, Cook TA, Wang TD. Irradiated costal cartilage in augmentation rhinoplasty. *Oper Techn Otolaryng.*
3. Rohrich RJ, Adams WP Jr. The boxy nasal tip: Classification and management based on alar cartilage suturing techniques. *Plast Reconstr Surg.* 2001 Jun;107(7):1849–1863.
4. Guyuron, Bahman RA. Nasal tip sutures part II: The interplay. *Plast Reconstr Surg.* 2003;112:1130.

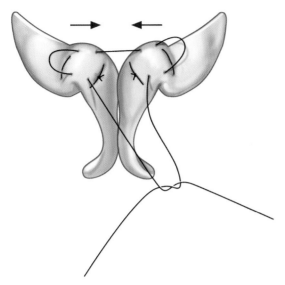

Figure 24-3. Intradomal and interdomal sutures to achieve nasal tip definition.

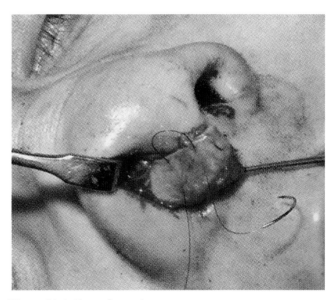

Figure 24-4. Lateral crural suture to convert a concave area into a convex one.

Chapter 25. Lower Lateral Cartilage Grafting Techniques

- *Indications*: Certain patients may have insufficiency of the lower lateral cartilage resulting in either functional or aesthetic abnormalities. In such cases, autogenous cartilage will provide adequate replacement or augmentation to deficient, weak, or deformed tip cartilage. Cartilage can be harvested from the septum (if available), ear, or costal margin for placement as a graft in these patients. In other patients, notching of the alar rim may be managed by placing a graft to span the area of the notch.
- *Assessment and markings*: Although there are no specific markings that need to be made, a thorough dimensional analysis of the patient's existing nasal tip projection and rotation should be performed. There are many tip grafts described in the literature, and the most useful and their indications will be described in this section.
- *Approach*: The tip region may be approached via either an open or a closed technique. The open approach will utilize a transcolumellar incision extended along each alar rim distal to the inferior edge of the lower lateral cartilages.
- *Technique*: The shield graft derives its name from its roughly triangular shape. It is used to provide definition and projection to the nasal tip (Figures 25-1 and 25-2). The shape and size of the graft are determined from the patient's anatomy. The length is roughly determined from the junction of the lobule and columella to a point just above the desired projection. The width at the inferior aspect is slightly narrower than that of the columella. The width at the superior aspect is determined so as not to produce too narrow or too boxy a tip.[1] If the graft is noted to be too angled, the edges should be beveled to minimize show. If too rigid, it can be softened by gentle crushing prior to being sutured into place.

- Additional tip grafts can be placed superior to the shield-type graft to further define the nasal tip and improve tip projection.[2] Several grafts have been described: cap graft (small graft placed between tip defining points), umbrella graft (vertical columellar strut combined with a horizontal onlay graft), onlay tip graft (horizontal graft placed over alar domes), and others. These are all variants of cartilage grafts placed on the nasal tip in slightly different locations.[3]
- One of the more common grafts placed within the lower lateral cartilages is the columellar strut (Figure 25-3). It can be used to increase tip projection, decrease tip rotation, straighten deflected medial lower lateral crura, and simply provide increased caudal nasal support. The graft is fabricated in the shape of a long rectangle. The base may or may not rest on the anterior nasal spine. Some surgeons avoid contact of the inferior aspect of the graft with the nasal spine to avoid any undesirable feeling or clicking of the graft.[4] The columellar strut is sutured in place between the medial crura of the lower lateral cartilages to provide tip support. The superior aspect may extend slightly above the domes of the middle crura to increase or maintain nasal tip projection but should not put excessive tension on the skin overlying the nasal tip. If a large degree of tip projection is desired, the strut can be secured to the anterior maxilla just off midline of the anterior nasal spine. A 0.035-in K-wire can be inserted longitudinally into about three quarters the length of the graft. The free end of the K-wire is trimmed and placed into a 12-mm hole drilled just off midline adjacent to the anterior nasal spine. With the K-wire inserted into the drilled hole, the graft is secure and can be bent into its desired position, making it an excellent anchorage point off which the surgeon can secure the tip.[5]

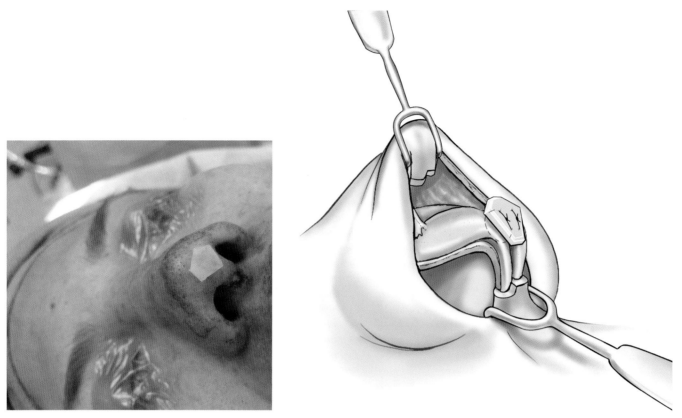

Figure 25-1. Position of the shield graft.

Figure 25-2. Shield graft.

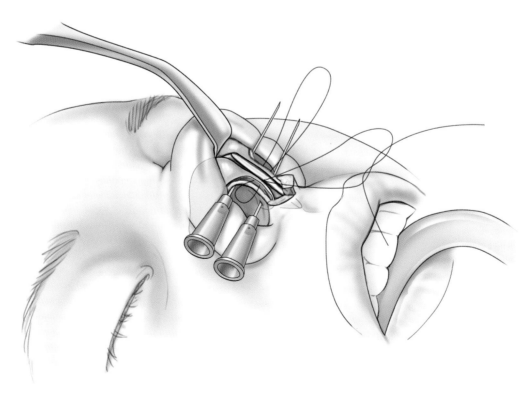

Figure 25-3. Twenty-five–gauge needles used to facilitate placement of a columellar strut graft.

○ In the setting of external valve collapse—either uni- or bilateral, alar batten grafts can be positioned over dorsal surface of one or both lower lateral cartilages (Figures 25-4 and 25-5). The grafts need not be completely rigid but should provide resistance to the negative inspiratory pressure created during inhalation. Batten grafts usually measure 10 mm to 15 mm in length and 3 mm to 4 mm in width. If bilateral grafts are to be used, they should be symmetrical. With isolated problems of the external valve, a closed approach is sufficient. The superior border of the lower lateral cartilage is identified and a subcutaneous pocket is created by dissecting in a plane just above the surface of the cartilage.[6]

○ An alar rim graft is used to treat or prevent alar retraction or collapse. These grafts are placed just above and parallel to the alar rim. A small incision is made and the grafts are inserted through a subcutaneous pocket. In cases of severe alar retraction, a lateral crural strut graft is usually more effective and can be used in addition to or in place of an alar rim graft.[7]

○ An alar spreader graft is a rectangular graft that is placed between the deep side of the lower lateral cartilages and the vestibular skin. This graft is sutured to each lateral crus and serves as a deep strut to maintain distance between the alar domes. This is useful to treat a pinched tip and also improves internal and external nasal valve function.[8]

○ Lateral crural onlay grafts are used to treat alar contour deformities from intact, but deformed lateral crura. They are placed over the lateral crura in a superficial manner. If done bilaterally, they need to be symmetric. Because irregularities may become apparent, the graft requires meticulous beveling or peripheral morsellization.[9]

• *Postoperative management*: Internally, nasal packing can be placed in the anterior portion of the vestibule if temporary support to the alar margin is desired. Externally, a single Steri-strip placed down one sidewall, across the columella, and back up the other sidewall suffices as a dressing to hold the repositioned columella in place.

• *Pitfalls*:
  ○ A visible tip graft should be avoided at all costs. Placement of semirigid cartilage grafts beneath a thin skin envelope will lead to eventual unnatural show of the margins of the graft. If this is encountered, the graft should be removed before closing the incision and gradually reduced to the point where support is maintained but not at the expense of visibility.

• *Tips*:
  ○ Precise modification of the tip is perhaps better performed via an external approach, although many surgeons can achieve success via a closed approach. If the latter is chosen, the pocket for a tip graft should be minimized to prevent migration. In the open approach, careful placement and suturing of the grafts into place is of paramount importance.
  ○ If the patient has thin skin and concern exists for eventual graft show, a thin piece of fascia from the temporal region may be used to cover the reconstructed, composite tip.

REFERENCES

1. Kamer FM, Churukian MM. Shield graft for the nasal tip. *Arch Otolaryngol.* 1984;110(9):608–610.
2. Sheen JH, Sheen AP. *Aesthetic Rhinoplasty.* 2nd ed. St. Louis, MO: Mosby; 1987:506–529.
3. Gunter JP, Landecker A, Cochran CS. Frequently used grafts in rhinoplasty: Nomencland and analysis. *Plast Reconstr Surg.* 2006;118:14e.
4. Gunter JP. Personal approaches: Gunter's approach. In JP Gunter RJ Rohrich, Adams WP Jr. In: *Dallas Rhinoplasty: Nasal Surgery by the Masters.* 1st ed. St Louis, MO: Quality Medical Publishing; 2002:1049.
5. Gunter JP, Clark CP, Friedman RM. Internal stabilization of autogenous rib cartilage grafts in rhinoplasty: A barrier to cartilage warping. *Plast Reconstr Surg.* 1997;100:161.
6. Toriumi D, Josen J, Weinberges M. Use of alar batten grafts for correction of nasal valve collapse. *Arch Otolaryngol Head and Neck Surg.* 1997;123:802.
7. Rohrich RJ, Raniere J, Ha R. The alar contour graft: Correction and prevention of alar rim deformities in rhinoplasty. *Plast Reconstr Surg.* 2002;109:2495.
8. Gunter JP, Rohrich RJ. Correction of the pinched nasal tip with alar spreader grafts. *Plast Reconstr Surg.* 1992; 90:821.
9. Watson D, Toriumi DM. Structural grafting in secondary rhinoplasty. In: Gunter JP, Rohrich RJ, Adams WP Jr. *Dallas Rhinoplasty: Nasal Surgery by the Masters,* 1st ed. St Louis, MO: Quality Medical Publishing; 2002:705.

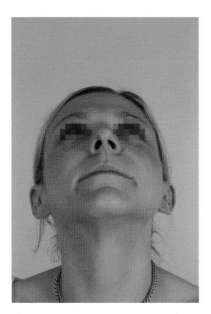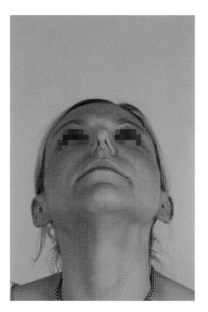

Figure 25-4. Worm's eye view of a patient demonstrating external value collapse with inspiration.

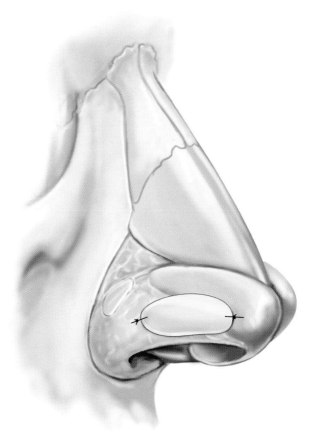

Figure 25-5. Alar batten graft.

Chapter 26. Lengthening the Short Nose

- *Indications*: The short nose can be a challenging problem to fix (Figure 26-1). As mentioned in previous sections, manipulation of the radix may aid in changing nasal length. A shallow radix can be deepened, which will move the nasion superiorly and therefore, increase nasal length. Additionally, if the superior dorsum of the nose is low, a graft will also cause the nasion to move superiorly and increase nasal length. If the tip is over-rotated, decreasing tip rotation will increase the length of the nose. However, when the nasion is normal or in cases of a severely short nose, additional procedures are necessary.
- *Markings*: No markings are necessary, but careful analysis and treatment planning is necessary to achieve an optimal result.
- *Approach*: A graduated approach to nasal lengthening is recommended. Because the soft tissue will need to allow the tip to rotate in an inferior direction, wide skin undermining is performed.
- *Technique*: The lower lateral cartilages are released from their attachments to the upper lateral cartilages and the caudal septum. The mobile tip is now rotated in an inferior direction.[1] A septal extension graft may be used to stabilize the tip in its new position. In more severe cases, aggressive techniques can be performed like tongue-in-groove septal extension grafts. A cartilage graft is shaped into three pieces: two septal extension grafts and a columellar strut graft. The septal extension grafts are placed at the dorsa septum and extend anteriorly between the middle crura. A columellar strut is also placed. The columellar strut can be sutured to the cantilevered extension grafts to fix the tip in its desired position (Figure 26-2).[2] For additional projection, tip grafts may be placed. The dorsal hump may become apparent as tip rotation decreases.[3] The beneficial effects of nasal lengthening can create unintended negative effects on other aspects of the nose. Derotation and lengthening of the tip will lower the nasal tip relative to the dorsum. Dorsal reduction can be done, if indicated, after the tip is in its new position. Additionally, alar flaring may occur with decreased tip rotation and if so, will need to be addressed.
- *Pitfalls*:
  - This technique frequently requires sizable amounts of cartilage, and a rib harvest is frequently necessary for this reason.
  - The cartilage may warp compromising the result.
- *Tips*:
  - Cartilage should be carved equally on both sides to avoid asymmetry.
  - Perichondrium should be removed from the graft material.
  - Undermining the skin should be wide enough to ensure that the cartilage complex will not be under tension in its new position.
  - .25 or .5 mm PDS foil may be used to reinforce grafts and reduce warping.

REFERENCES

1. Gunter JP, Rohrich RJ. Lengthening the aesthetically short nose. *Plast Reconstr Surg*. 1989;83:793.
2. Guyuron B, Varghai A. Lengthening the nose with a tongue and groove technique. *Plast Reconstr Surg*. 2003;111:1533.
3. Hamra S. Lengthening the foreshortened nose. *Plast Reconstr Surg*. 2001;108:547.

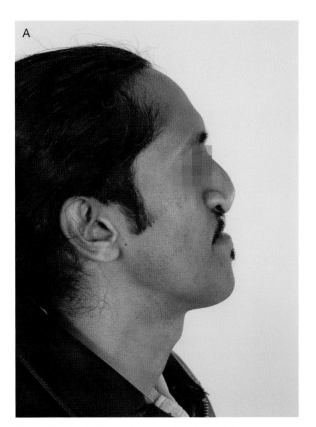 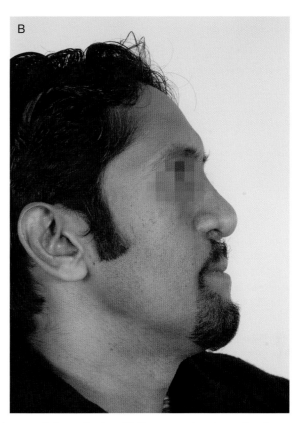

Figure 26-1. **A.** Lateral view of patient with short nose and decreased tip projection. **B.** Postoperative view of patient after nasal lengthening with anterior septal extension grafts and a columellar strut graft.

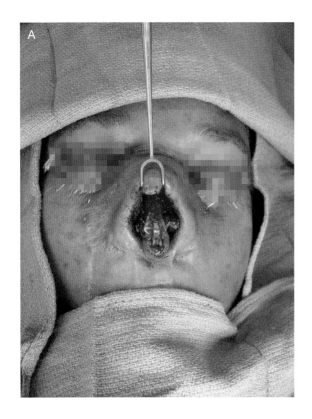

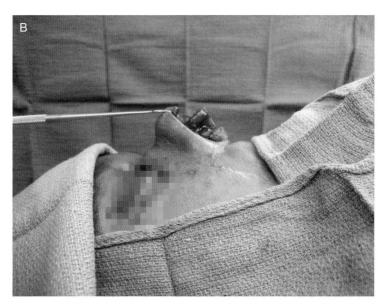

Figure 26-2. **A.** Frontal view of columellar strut graft sutured to anterior septal extension graft to increase nasal length and projection. **B.** The anterior septal extension graft is sutured to the superior border of the dorsal septum and extends anteriorly to give structural support to the columellar strut.

Chapter 27. Nasal Osteotomies: Width Manipulation

- *Indications*: Nasal osteotomies are indicated for narrowing wide lateral walls of the nose, closing an open roof deformity, or straightening the nasal bony framework in a deviated nose. Nasal osteotomies are frequently performed in rhinoplasty surgery. In fact, one study found that osteotomies were performed on over 95% of their patients (by comparison, a dorsal hump was removed on 84%).[1] These maneuvers are challenging because they are not directly visualized and often lack the control that is present with other interventions. Once osteotomized, the small nasal bones are not fixed as are other bones but are splinted from above and below in order to maintain the desired intraoperative position. In order for the surgeon to maintain control of the osteotomized segments, the procedure must be completed in a meticulous manner.
- *Markings*: Drawing the planned course of the osteotomy on the skin is often helpful since it may serve as a guide to follow with a finger palpating the tip of the osteotome. Remember that the low osteotomy does not begin in the nasal bone but rather on the maxilla.
- *Classifications*: The position of the osteotomy may be described by the starting and ending points along the piriform aperture and relative to the midline. A low osteotomy is positioned further off the midline while a high osteotomy is positioned more medially, or higher on the lateral nasal wall. Each type of osteotomy has an indication.[2]
  - A low-low osteotomy mobilizes a larger segment of lateral nasal wall and is used when mobilization of the bony roof is needed to correct a very wide nasal base or a large open roof deformity. The low-low osteotomy is also useful in patients with small nasal bones because it creates larger segments of bone to compensate for the scant nasal bone surface area. The low-low osteotomy also perhaps best mirrors the natural shape of the nasal bones (Figure 27-1).
  - A low-high osteotomy is used to correct a small open roof deformity or correct a medium-wide nasal base. Higher osteotomies may be preferable in the occasional patient with larger nasal bones to achieve better dorsal refinement (Figure 27-1).
  - *Double level osteotomies*: These are used when excessively convex lateral nasal walls are present or if lateral nasal deformities or asymmetries are present. Additionally, it can be useful in smoothing the transition from the cheek to the nasal sidewall when deformities exist.[3] The double osteotomies consist of two parallel osteotomies: one low-low and another more medial (higher) on the nasal wall. The order is important since performing the more lateral osteotomy first leaves an unattached and unstable piece of bone to cut secondarily.
  - *Medial osteotomies*: A medial osteotomy separates the nasal bones from one another in the midline (Figure 27-2). It is recommended when the dorsal aspect of the nose needs to be narrowed in isolation or in conjunction with the base of the nose where lateral osteotomies would also be required. Other indications are male patients with thicker bone in the region of the radix or patients with deviation of the nasal root who require mobilization and repositioning the nasal pyramid. The medial osteotomy is initiated at the lateral edge of the open roof deformity or proceeds in a lateral direction if no open roof deformity is present. It proceeds in a superolateral direction 15 degrees off the midline where a natural cleavage plane exists for the osteotomy.[4] This is easily marked on the patient as a line extending to a point halfway between the nasion and the medial canthus. The lateral nasal bone is then placed so that its superior edge gets tucked medially under the intact nasal bone. Any palpable edge can be smoothed with a rasp. If combined with a lateral osteotomy, it is important to leave about 2 mm to 5 mm of bone intact between the two superior ends of the osteotomies. The medial osteotomy with or without a lateral osteotomy is capable of narrowing the dorsum of the nose.[5]

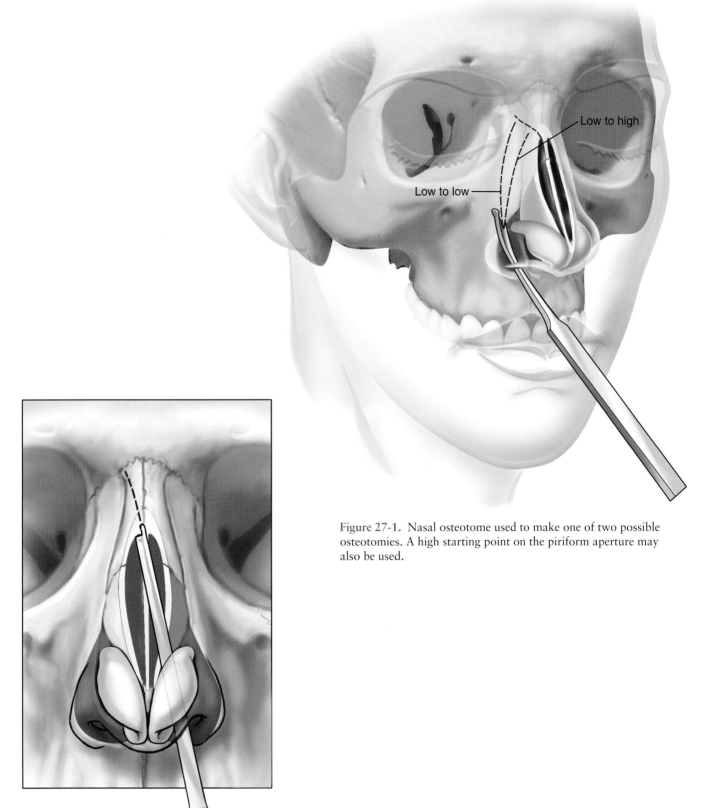

Figure 27-1. Nasal osteotome used to make one of two possible osteotomies. A high starting point on the piriform aperture may also be used.

Figure 27-2. Medial osteotomy.

- *Approaches*: There are several acceptable approaches for accessing the bony nasal vault for the purpose of performing a lateral nasal osteotomy: endonasal, percutaneous, and gingivobuccal. The surgeon should understand and be comfortable performing each even though he may have a preferred approach.
- *Techniques*: For the endonasal and gingivobuccal approaches, the osteotomy is often performed with a specialized, curved osteotome with a notched or guarded tip. A larger, bulbous side is ahead of the cutting edge and the shorter, sharper edge is closer to the cutting surface. The notched tip of the osteotome straddles the free inferior edge of the nasal bone with the larger side external to the bone, where it is palpable but has minimal chance of piercing the skin. The smaller tip stays inside the nasal bone. While injury to the mucosa is possible, this heals well and rarely causes a problem. A sharp 2-mm osteotome is typically recommended for the percutaneous approach. Lidocaine (1%) with 1:100,000 epinephrine should be injected into the lateral and medial nasal walls at least 7 minutes prior to the osteotomies in order to minimize bleeding and postoperative bruising.
  - *Endonasal approach*: A small incision is made within the lateral nasal vestibule to provide access to the inferior junction of the nasal bones with the frontal process of the maxilla. The location for the incision is identified by retracting laterally on the nasal sidewall to drape the mucosa over the underlying piriform aperture. The incision should be just large enough to allow introduction of the nasal osteotome. Through this incision, a narrow subcutaneous dissection with a Freer periosteal elevator along the external aspect of the nasal sidewall is performed. It is important to only dissect a tunnel just big enough to accommodate the osteotome in order to preserve as much of the soft tissue attachment to the osteotomized nasal wall as possible. The osteotome is then passed along the same tunnel of dissection. Again, the longer, blunted tip of the osteotome is left external to the nasal bone so that it may be palpated beneath the skin and not puncture the skin. The sharper tip is left inside the piriform aperture medial to the nasal bones. One can palpate the tip as the osteotomy proceeds, verifying the proper orientation as the osteotomy progresses. The incision can remain open or be loosely closed so that fluid may drain.
  - *Percutaneous approach*: A small, 2-mm osteotome is introduced through a small incision at the level of the inferior orbital rim. The technique is advantageous because it allows excellent control of the proposed line of fracture by its direct approach, minimizes subperiosteal dissection resulting in more stability and less dead space, and thus reduces postoperative edema and recovery time. A small stab incision just medial to the inferior orbital rim is made with a #11 blade or the osteotome itself can be used to penetrate the skin if it is sharp. Through this incision, a 2-mm osteotome is used, in a subperiosteal plane, to create a line of perforations along the nasal sidewall by angling the instrument superiorly and inferiorly (Figure 27-3). Again, skin markings of the proposed osteotomy may help guide the surgeon while the osteotomy progresses (Figure 27-4). The skin is shifted with the osteotome to maximize the reach of the single skin incision. The incision is closed with a Steri-strip postoperatively.[6] The percutaneous scars heal well and have not been found to present a problem.[7]

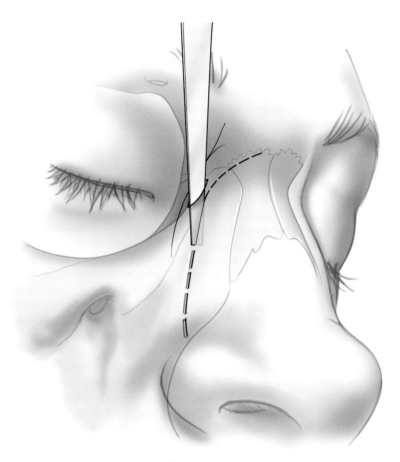

Figure 27-3. Schematic drawing of the percutaneous osteotomy technique.

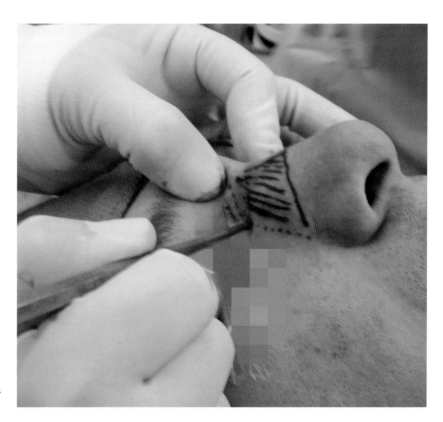

Figure 27-4. Intraoperative photograph demonstrating a percutaneous osteotomy. Nasal bones are indicated in purple.

○ *Gingivobuccal sulcus approach*: A small incision is made in the mucosa of the gingivobuccal sulcus in line with the proposed osteotomy (Figure 27-5). This may be done with electrocautery down to the bony surface of the maxilla to minimize bleeding. Similar to the above techniques, a tunnel is dissected along the piriform aperture and up to the level of the nasofrontal junction. Care is taken not to strip too much tissue or create too big a tunnel in order to preserve some soft tissue attachments to the nasal bones. While carrying the dissection superiorly, the takeoff of the nasal bones should be appreciated since it is below this level along the frontal process of the maxilla that the osteotomy commences (Figure 27-6). The gingivobuccal approach is perhaps the most direct approach to the nasal bones. Controlled advancement of the osteotome with the mallet is performed similar to the endonasal approach (Figure 27-7). The incision is either left open or loosely closed to facilitate fluid drainage.

• *Postoperative*: The percutaneous and gingivobuccal sulcus incisions may be left open, while the intranasal incision is closed with one or two sutures. The percutaneous site may be covered with a small adhesive strip. Internal and external support is usually indicated to hold the nasal bones in position as they heal back to the frontal bone and maxilla. Internal splinting is achieved with Vaseline gauze or resorbable foam packing. External support is achieved with a tape dressing beneath a rigid splint. The splint may be fabricated from multiple layers of plaster cut into a rough trapezoidal shape, thermoplastic polymer, or padded aluminum. If the nasal bones are not secure in their new position, it is preferable to use a splint that can be easily applied to its desired dimensions with little pressure on the nasal bones. Either plaster or a thermoplastic material works well in this situation. In such cases, the splint is generally left in place for 10 to 14 days to allow healing and remind the patient to avoid any potentially harmful contact. Careful removal is facilitated by swabs soaked in acetone or other adhesive-removing solution.

• *Pitfalls*:
  ○ Not every patient is a candidate for nasal bone osteotomy. Older patients with thin bones may not produce a clean osteotomy line and patients who wear heavy eyeglasses may depress the nasal bones farther than desired.
  ○ Laceration of the skin is certainly a possibility if the sharper side of the osteotome faces outward to minimize mucosal injury (not recommended). For the percutaneous approach, care should be taken to avoid injury to the angular artery that courses through the nasal sidewall. Local anesthesia with epinephrine should be injected in the area before making the skin incision and the scalpel should pass only superficially through the skin.

○ The starting position for the lateral osteotomy should not be below the level of the inferior turbinate. Too low a takeoff will include that part of the frontal process of the maxilla, which serves as support for the most lateral portion of the lower lateral cartilage and thus integrity of the external nasal valve.
○ At the lateral junction of the upper and lower lateral cartilages, just medial to the nasal bones, care should be taken to avoid injury to the triangle of soft tissue that supports the external nasal valve.
○ An osteotomy that is too high on the nasal bones may result in formation of either a visible or palpable ledge. It may be avoided either with a lower osteotomy on the maxilla or a double osteotomy. Correction of the postoperative ledge may be addressed with a secondary osteotomy lower on the maxilla to soften the step-off between the nasal bone and the maxilla. A bony spike in the region of the medial canthus may be the superior edge of the infractured nasal bone.

• *Tips*:
  ○ Preoperatively, the surgeon should have a reasonable estimation of the size of the nasal bones and decide on the most ideal path for the planned osteotomy.
  ○ In creating the subcutaneous tunnel along the lateral nasal sidewall, care should be taken to avoid devascularizing the free bony segment and prevent unintended malposition by preserving some of the lateral soft tissue attachment.
  ○ Intranasally, confirm the position of the inferior turbinate as a starting point for the lateral osteotomy and osteotomize from this point cephalad.
  ○ As the osteotome is advanced superiorly, the angle of the instrument should be controlled and the target point medial to the medial canthus kept on line.

REFERENCES

1. Ponsky D, Eshraghi Y, Guyuron B. The frequency of surgical maneuvers during open rhinoplasty. *Plast Reconstr Surg.* 2010 Jul;126(1):240–244.
2. Rohrich R, Krueger JK, Adams WP, Hollier LH. Achieving consistency in the lateral nasal osteotomy during rhinoplasty: An external perforated technique. *Plast Reconstr Surg.* 108: 2122, 2001.
3. Westreich RW, Lawson W. Perforating double lateral osteotomy. *Arch Facial Plast Surg.* 2005 Jul–Aug;7(4):257–260.
4. Tardy ME, Toriumi DM, Hecht DA. Philosophy and principles of rhinoplasty. In: Papel ID, ed. *Facial and Plastic Reconstructive Surgery.* New York: Thieme; 2002:384–389.
5. Gruber R, Chang T, Kahn D, et al. Broad nasal bone reduction: An algorithm for osteotomies. *Plast Reconstr Surg.* 2007;119:1044.
6. Rohrich R, Krueger JK, Adams WP, Hollier LH. Achieving consistency in the lateral nasal osteotomy during rhinoplasty: An external perforated technique. *Plast Reconstr Surg.* 2001;108:2122.
7. Gryskiewicz J. Visible scars from percutaneous osteotomies. *Plast Reconstr Surg.* 2005;116:1771.

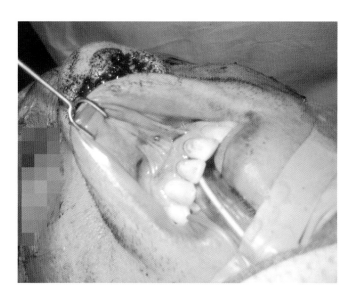

Figure 27-5. Exposure of the gingivobuccal sulcus for dissection of osteotomy plane.

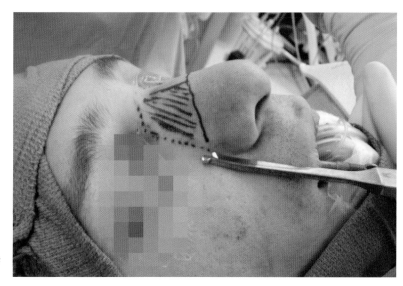

Figure 27-6. Course of the osteotome along the frontal process of the maxilla.

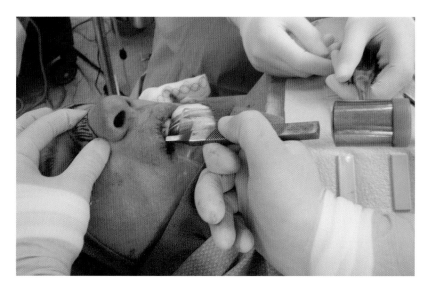

Figure 27-7. Osteotome positioned within the gingivobuccal sulcus and advanced superiorly with gentle tapping with a mallet.

Chapter 28. Alar Base Modification

- *Indications*: The alar base includes the alar rims as they begin medially at the tip and columella and curve laterally to end at the attachments to the cheek. Ideally, the alar base of the nose should approximate an equilateral triangle with a slight degree of convexity at the alar cheek junction (Figure 28-1). It should provide adequate support to prevent collapse of the external nasal valve and demonstrate minimal scarring. Each has a cutaneous outer portion and an inner vestibular portion with a greater or lesser amount of intervening soft tissue. Preoperatively, the frontal view should identify the width of the alar base (Figure 28-2). Each side should be carefully examined in tandem, as well as separate from one another. In general, the alar bases are slightly wider than the distance between the medial and lateral canthi and should not extend past a vertical line dropped from the medial canthus. Excessive flaring or convexity of the alar bases should be documented if present. The lateral view will identify the cranial-caudal position of the alar base. It will also highlight the position of the alar rim and the columella separately and as they relate to one another (this will be examined separately in the following section). Finally, the basal view will identify the size of the nostril openings and the degree of flaring on each side. The long axis of the nostril should be at a 50- degree to 60-degree angle off a vertical line through the columella, and the nostril to tip proportion should be about 60:40 to 55:45. With careful inspection and palpation, the examiner should judge the quality of the skin and underlying soft tissue. The outer cutaneous surface should be considered separate from the inner vestibular surface. Any external or internal scarring of the skin and/or mucosa should be noted. In some patients, the nostril size and shape are adequate, but the overall inter-alar width is excessive on account of an excessively thick alar rim. In these patients, resection of a greater width of the cutaneous surface versus the vestibular surface might be indicated. Antero-posterior, oblique, lateral, and most importantly, worm's eye views on preoperative photographs are critical to highlight the characteristics of the alar complex.

- *Markings*: The preoperative markings are important to ensure the appropriate amount of tissue is resected. In patients with more malleable skin and soft tissue, the alar base can be gently grasped and advanced towards the cheek to give the surgeon a rough idea of the amount of resection that is both needed and tolerable without undue tension. Calipers should be used to carefully measure the amount of tissue to be excised (Figure 28-3). Certainly, in instances where there is an unequal nostril size, differing amounts of tissue can be resected. Two curvilinear lines are marked on the cutaneous surface perpendicular to the alar rim. The lines will converge over the surface of the nose before advancing onto the nasal sidewall. They should not extend superior to the alar crease to avoid injury to the lateral nasal vessels.[1] The incision should be made 1 mm above the alar-cheek junction to preserve the curvature of the rim and avoid having the scar fall within the alar crease. Variable amounts of lining skin and mucosa can be removed.

- *Technique*: Several alar rim deformities can been encountered. Their characteristics and treatment are discussed below.
  - The ala may appear unnaturally concave when it bends medially and can have several etiologies, including interruption of the lower lateral cartilage, improper placement of a tip graft that extends lateral to the dome, or resection of the lower lateral cartilage. The concavity is best treated with the insertion of an alar rim graft. The graft can be placed through a small incision into a subcutaneous pocket. The pocket can be dissected with iris scissors and advanced along the alar rim.
  - The ala may also appear convex as a result of either an excessively convex lower lateral cartilage or thick alar tissue. When the problem is related to convex lower lateral cartilage, it may be treated with either intradomal sutures or lateral crural spanning sutures depending on where the convexity is located. If the convexity is due to excessive thickness of alar tissue, a small elliptical incision can be made as close to the medial nostril rim as possible. This allows removal of skin and subcutaneous tissue to thin the ala.[2]

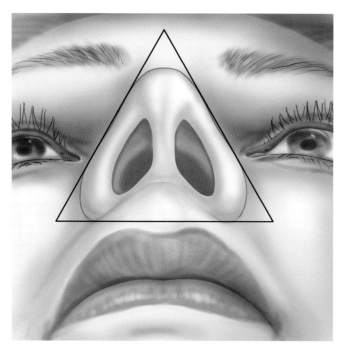

Figure 28-1. Worm's eye view demonstrating the roughly equilateral triangle of the alar base.

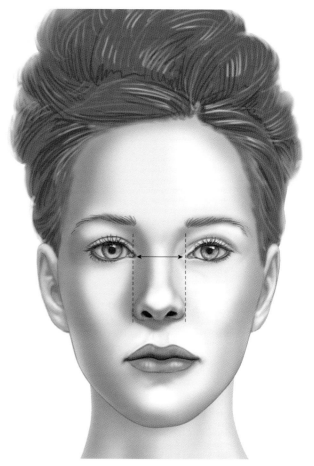

Figure 28-2. The alar width should approximate the distance between the medial canthi.

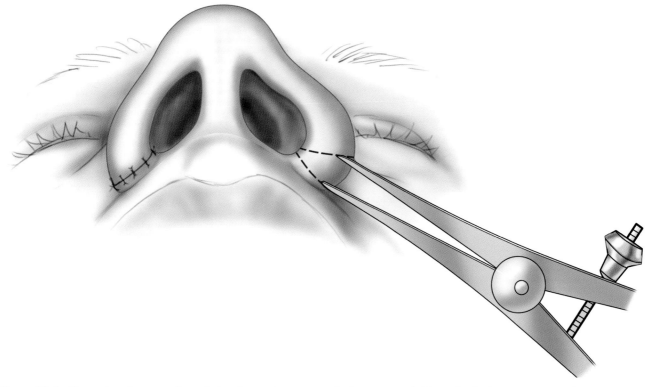

Figure 28-3. Measuring the contralateral alar rim so that symmetrical amounts of skin and soft tissue are removed.

○ When resecting part of the alar base, two surfaces are potentially involved: the cutaneous and vestibular surfaces. Excision of the cutaneous surface will only affect the contour of the alar lobule but not nostril circumference. In contrast, excision of the vestibular skin will reduce the aperture of the nostril. The surgeon must assess the degree to which each should be altered independently. In a patient with a large alar lobule and normal nostril area, the lobule should be reduced without the vestibular skin. In a patient that exhibits both a large lobule and nostril, a wedge that includes both cutaneous and vestibular skin may be removed. To start, nearly parallel curvilinear incisions are made at the most lateral margin of the alar rim with a #11 scalpel blade as previously marked. The alar lobule may be steadied with the opposite hand by pinching the rim more medially. The opposite index finger can palpate the vestibular surface so that the knife approaches this inner surface but does not pass through it if the vestibular skin is to remain intact. As noted, a 1-mm edge of lateral alar rim should be spared to preserve the curvature of the rim and improve the appearance of the scar. If a full-thickness resection is required, the incision into the vestibule should cross the nostril edge at a right angle rather than an acute, oblique angle. This leaves a small triangular flap medially, which serves to minimize unnatural notching in the corner of the nostril.[3] The incisions are deepened to the level of the mucosa (or through the mucosa) so that a wedge of skin and subcutaneous tissue (and mucosa) is excised (Figure 28-4). Careful hemostasis is obtained and the edges approximated in layers. One or two deep absorbable sutures should be placed to reduce tension on the repair and 6-0 nylon sutures should be placed to approximate the skin edges and removed early to minimize suture marks on the skin edges (Figure 28-5). If mucosa was included in the resection, it is best reapproximated first with absorbable sutures, such as 4-0 or 5-0 chromic gut, followed by subcutaneous tissue and finally skin. Following resection on a single side, the worm's eye view will highlight the desired change in nostril size and shape.

○ If the alar base is cranially displaced and medial translocation alone is not shown to drop its position sufficiently, an elliptical wedge of skin at the alar base–upper lip junction may be resected. After freeing the underlying soft tissue attachments of the alar base, the inferior margin is sutured to the new superior aspect of the upper lip with both deep absorbable sutures as well as cutaneous sutures. Similarly, if the alar base is caudally displaced, an elliptical resection of mucosa may be performed within the vestibular lining just above the alar rim to raise the base as the edges are reapproximated.

○ If the alar base is laterally displaced, release of the base and addition of a cinch suture may be indicated to narrow the alar complex. This may be done via a gingivobuccal sulcus incision to allow access to the piriform aperture and release of the deep soft tissue attachments with a periosteal elevator. To provide closer approximation of the alar bases, deep bites into the tissue of each ala are taken with 3-0 PDS suture. Two of these sutures are used and are tied so that each ala has a deep knot at its side. The suture should be initially cinched into the desired position with little if any overcorrection.[4]

○ In rare instances, the alar complex is wide due solely to a thick alar lobule and the nostril size is deficient. A rim incision is made close to the apex of the nostril internally, and an ellipse of tissue is excised followed by a coring out of thick fibrous tissue. The results of this operation are subtle and it takes time for the edema to resolve.[5]

• *Postoperative management*: Antibiotic ointment can be applied to the suture line in the immediate postoperative period since a dressing in this specific area may occlude the nostril and be difficult to keep in place. Non-dissolvable sutures should be removed within a week to avoid undesirable scarring.

• *Pitfalls*:
  ○ Excessive resection of tissue at the alar base can lead to obliteration of the normal curvature of the alar rim. Inspection of the nose from a worm's eye view would reveal an unnatural straightening of the alar margin and too acute an angle at the nostril sill.
  ○ Scarring in the region of the alar base is more noticeable than in other areas of the nose and can be a telltale sign of surgery.

• *Tips*:
  ○ Care should be taken in designing the appropriate incisions. They should leave a small cuff of skin on the lateral cheek and not extend superiorly past the alar crease. Fine caliber absorbable sutures or permanent sutures that are removed early should also be used.
  ○ Caution dictates that the more internal lining is removed, the more unnatural postoperative straightening of the alar rim will occur. Therefore, care should be taken in not designing the internal resection margins too widely.
  ○ Err on conservatism. This is a procedure that can be revised in the office under local anesthesia if more resection is required.

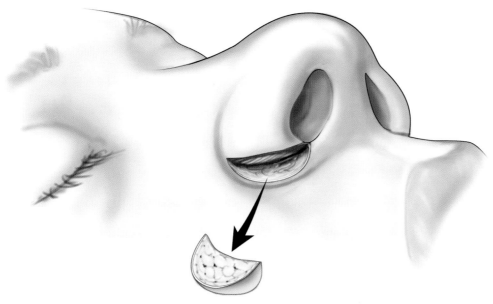

Figure 28-4. Removal of skin and soft tissue without mucosa.

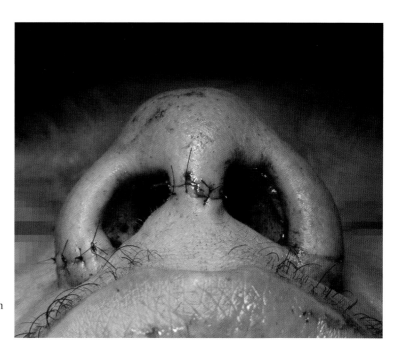

Figure 28-5. Worm's eye photograph following resection of the right alar base and before the left to highlight the change in the appearance of the nose.

REFERENCES

1. Guyuron B. Alar rim deformities. *Plast Reconstr Surg.* 2001;107:856.
2. Matarasso A. Alar rim excision: A method of thinning bulky nostrils. *Plast Reconstr Surg.* 2001;108:1425.
3. Rohrich RJ, Gunter JP, Friedman RM. Nasal tip blood supply: An anatomic study validating the safety of the transcolumellar incision in rhinoplasty. *Plast Reconstr Surg.* 1999;5:795.
4. Sheen JH. Alar resection and grafting. In: Gunter JP, Rohrich RJ, Adams WP, eds. *Dallas Rhinoplasty.* St. Louis, MO: Quality Medical Publishing; 2002:917.
5. Gruber R, Freeman M, Hsv C. Nasal, et al. Nasal base reduction: A treatment algorithm including alar release with medialization. *Plast Reconstr Surg.* 2009;123:716.

Chapter 29. Alar-Columellar Relationship Modification

- *Indications*: In order to evaluate the alar-columellar relationship, the surgeon must understand the ideal aesthetic norm for this anatomic relationship. From the lateral view, the ideal amount of columellar show has been described as about 2 mm to 3 mm.[1] A line drawn from the apex of the nostril to its nadir should divide the nostril in equal halves. A retracted ala is present when the alar rim is greater than 2 mm from this line (Figure 29-1) and a hanging ala occurs when the ala is within 1.5 mm of this line (Figure 29-2). Likewise a hanging columella occurs when the columella is greater than 2 mm from the long axis of the nostril (Figure 29-3), and a retracted columella occurs when the columella is within 1.5 mm of the long axis of the nostril[2] (Figure 29-4). It is important to remember that there may be a combination of both alar and columellar abnormalities that contribute to the deformity. Proper treatment begins with identifying the etiology and specifically addressing the cause.

- *Markings*: There are no specific markings on the patient that need to be made for planning. However, the precise relationship between the alar rim and the columella is best evaluated on a standard lateral photograph, and a clear acetate overlay allows measurements to be made that aid in diagnosis.

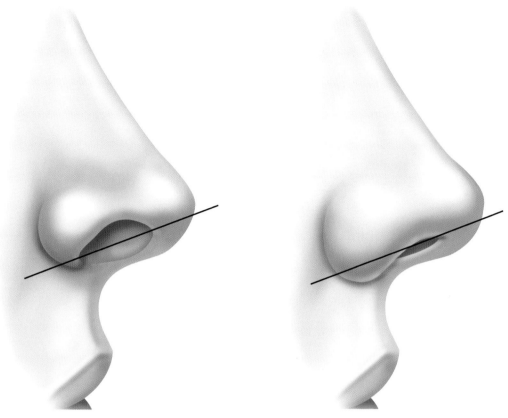

Figure 29-1. Retracted alar rim—Alar margin >2 mm from line.

Figure 29-2. Hanging alar rim—Alar margin within 1.5 mm of line.

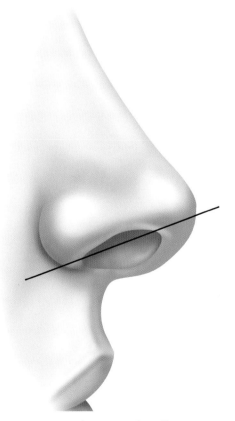

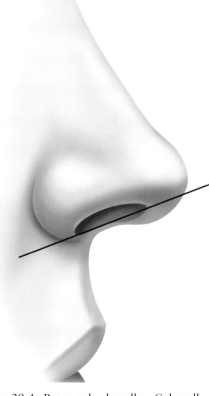

Figure 29-3. Overhanging columella—Columella >2 mm from line.

Figure 29-4. Retracted columella—Columella within 1.5 mm of line.

- *Technique*:
  - Several treatment options have been described for patients with excess columellar show due to a retracted alar rim and a normally positioned columella. An alar batten graft may help for minor retractions less than 1.5 mm. Alar batten grafts work better in primary rhinoplasties than in secondary rhinoplasties and may require additional support from a lateral crural strut graft in the scarred secondary rhinoplasty patient.[3] For larger degrees of alar retraction, a composite graft may be indicated. The internal surface of the rim is incised along the inferior aspect of the lower lateral cartilages similar to a standard rim incision. With gentle spreading of the soft tissues, the alar rim should rotate inferiorly to diminish the amount of lateral columellar exposure. The resultant opening is then filled with a graft of relatively stiff tissue, such as palatal mucosa, a combination of septal cartilage and mucosa, or a composite graft of conchal cartilage and skin. The graft is sutured to the periphery of the wound with 5-0 chromic sutures. A third option has been described by Guyuron.[4] A V-Y flap is designed with its apex at the superior internal nostril mucosa directly above the retraction. This incision needs to be incorporated into an open rhinoplasty incision so the V-Y flap's blood supply is not interrupted. A large inverted "V" flap is dissected internally above the retracted ala. It is raised so that the wide part of the "V" is the alar border, and the flap is freely dissected to the alar margin. This maneuver should release the alar retraction and the advanced "V" tissue is now set into its new location. A cartilage graft can be placed under this flap to maintain integrity of the alar rim. The resulting superior interior defect is closed in a V-Y fashion.
  - For patients with excess show due to a hanging columella and a normally positioned alar rim, resection of the medial footplates of the columella, the caudal septum, or both should correct the problem. For defects due to a combination of retracted alar rim and overhanging columella, both deformities should be individually addressed.[5]
  - Conversely, if columellar exposure is diminished and noted to be due to a low hanging alar rim, an incision may be made inside the alar rim and an ellipse of vestibular skin removed. This will elevate the alar rim and improve the amount of columellar show.

  - If the etiology is a retracted columella in the presence of normal alar rim position, augmentation of the caudal septum can be performed. A cartilage graft positioned at the inferior edge of the caudal septum between the medial crura of the lower lateral cartilages will push the columella inferiorly and normalize the degree of show. Again, for defects due to a combination of a low alar rim and a retracted columella, each problem should be addressed separately.
- *Postoperative management*: A small packing of petroleum gauze should be left in the vestibule for a day or two, and a tape dressing should be placed across the columella for initial support. If not absorbable, the pack is removed in 24 to 48 hours to minimize the risk of infection.
- *Pitfalls*:
  - The most obvious complications include either under- or overcorrection of the alar rim position. If unilateral, the normal side should be used for comparison. If bilateral, correction should achieve roughly 2 mm of columellar show on lateral view.
- *Tips*:
  - The exact cause of the alar deformity should be carefully determined prior to surgery so that the appropriate intervention is employed.
  - If a graft is required to improve the alar-columellar relationship, slight overcorrection may be advised to combat normal postoperative graft contraction.
  - All attempts should be made to minimize the causes of graft loss, including shear, hematoma, and/or seroma formation in the postoperative period.

REFERENCES

1. Sheen JH. *Aesthetic Rhinoplasty*. St Louis, MO: Mosby; 1978.
2. Gunter JP, Rohrich RJ, Friedman RM. Classification and correction of alar-columellar discrepancies in rhinoplasty. *Plast Reconstr Surg*. 1996;97:643.
3. Rohrich R, Raniere J, Ha R. The alar contour graft: Correction and prevention of alar rim deformities in rhinoplasty. *Plast Reconstr Surg*. 2002;109:2495.
4. Guyuron B. Alar rim deformities. *Plast Reconstr Surg*. 2001;107:856.
5. Matarasso A, Greer SE, Longaker MT. The true hanging columella: Simplified diagnosis and treatment using a modified direct approach. *Plast Reconstr Surg*. 2000;106:469.

Chapter 30. Septal Modification

- *Indications*: Some deflection of the nasal septum in any plane is likely present in most patients. Those with significant deviation of the septum are candidates for septoplasty since deviation of the septum limits airflow at the level of the internal nasal valve. Obstruction of 50% to 60% of the anterior and inferior aspect of the airway generally leads to symptoms of obstruction. The diagnosis is made by careful internal examination with a nasal speculum and an adequate light source. At times, the deviation may be symptomatic by impeding airflow through one or both nostrils. Preoperatively, the nature of the deviation should be identified. Deflection of the septum can be simply in one plane, such as the anterior-posterior direction or superior-inferior direction, or in a combination of planes. The patient should be questioned about prior manipulation of the septum and evidence sought on physical examination. Often a scar will be noted on one or more sides of the septal mucosa to indicate prior intervention. A cotton-tipped application can be used to gently palpate the septum if there is concern that portions were previously removed or damaged. Cartilage that has been removed and replaced as a graft usually does not retain its earlier pliability.
- *Markings*: No external markings are necessary to plan one's approach to the nasal septum. The extent of the septum should be appreciated so that 1 cm of dorsal and caudal cartilage is preserved as supporting elements of the remaining septum. Depending upon one's internal approach, the proposed lateral mucosal incision may be drawn 1 cm from the caudal edge through the right nostril if the surgeon is standing on the right side of the operating room table.
- *Approach*: The septal cartilage may be harvested laterally through the nostril or caudally between the crura of the lower lateral cartilages. In either instance, both a topical and a submucosal vasoconstrictive agent should be used. Topically, oxymetazoline or cocaine is commonly used. The former is delivered by aerosolized spray while the latter may be dispensed as a 4% solution into a small cup and soaked into 1-in by 6-in cotton pledgets. To minimize absorption, the pledgets should be gently wrung out. These are then packed into the nose (two to three per side) after the nasal hairs are trimmed and before the face is prepped. Additionally, a dilute solution of epinephrine (1:200,000) may be injected submucosally on either side of the septum before beginning the harvest to further minimize bleeding as well as provide hydrodissection of the mucosa off the underlying cartilage. When a lateral approach is chosen, an incision may be made one centimeter from the caudal edge of the septum. This may be delineated by gently deflecting the columella to the left to identify the most inferior aspect of the septum. The incision should be made through the mucosa and perichondrium initially. Dissection then proceeds carefully along the cartilage with a Freer or cottle elevator. Leaving 1 cm of intact septum dorsally and caudally, the septal cartilage is traversed with the sharp end of the cottle elevator or a scalpel. This allows access for contralateral mucosal elevation from the septum. Care is taken to not violate the opposite mucosa to prevent fistula formation (Figure 30-1). This may be difficult if there is significant deflection of the septum either towards or away from the surgeon. Dissection should continue posteriorly to the perpendicular plate of the ethmoid and inferiorly to the vomer and anterior nasal spine (Figure 30-2). The caudal 1-cm margin of septum should be left intact to prevent collapse.
- *Technique*: Manipulation of the septum is then performed to achieve/restore straightness and thus improves airflow.

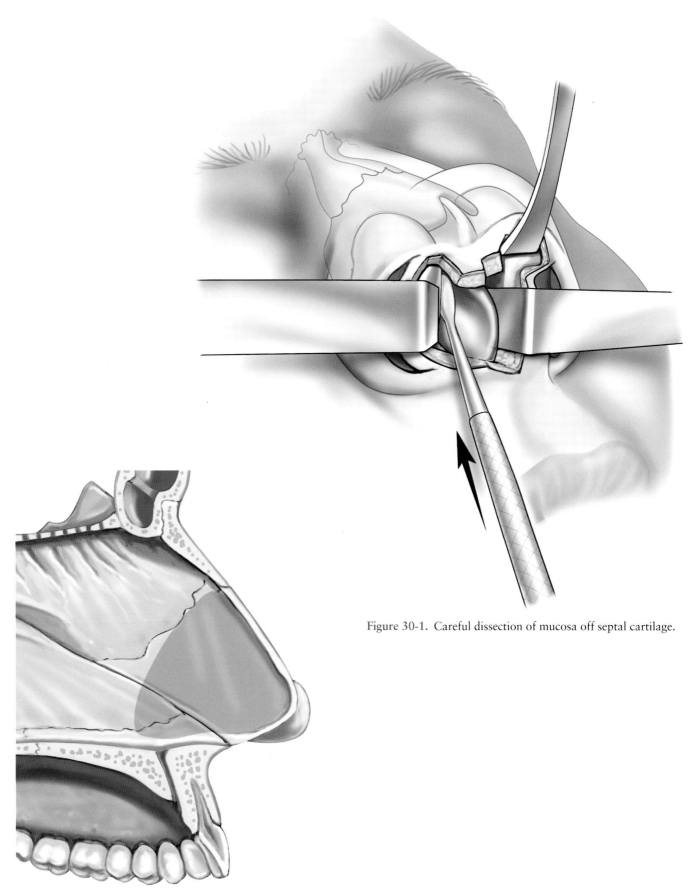

Figure 30-1. Careful dissection of mucosa off septal cartilage.

Figure 30-2. Extent of septal dissection.

○ If the septum is minimally deflected, it may be scored on the concave side to weaken it and facilitate bending (Figures 30-3 and 30-4). If it is moderately deflected, it may be incised at several levels to create a fan-like structure that is weaker than the deflected one. If severely deflected, a portion may be removed and either left out or softened by gentle crushing and replaced (Figure 30-5).

○ Closure of the septal mucosa should include dissolvable sutures to re-approximate the edges as well as mattress sutures to re-approximate the right and left sides if cartilage is removed. In this way, accumulation of fluid and blood into the potential space is minimized.

• *Postoperative management*: Following harvest of septal cartilage, the two leaves of mucosa should be re-approximated with absorbable mattress sutures. Some surgeons opt to pack the nostrils to further minimize the chance of fluid collecting beneath the mucosa. If nonabsorbable Vaseline gauze is used for packing, the patient should be placed on antibiotics to minimize the possibility of developing bacteremia and resultant toxic shock syndrome. A similar plan should be used for silicone tubes surrounded by absorptive material. Dissolvable Gelfoam may similarly be used for packing, but does not need to be removed.

• *Pitfalls*:
○ If dissection around the septum is too limited, injury to the mucosa is more likely with introduction of instruments to harvest the cartilage, such as a Ballenger knife.

○ Perforations of the mucosa overlying the septum may lead to persistent fistulae if they are opposite a mucosal defect. The best means of treatment is prevention. Care should be taken to slowly dissect the mucoperiosteum off the septal cartilage cognizant that unrecognized prior trauma to the septum might have led to areas of unnatural adherence.

○ Hematomas or seromas may form in areas between the mucosal leaves where cartilage was removed. To minimize this complication, one or more mattress sutures should be passed across the remaining intact mucosa to obliterate any potential dead space.

• *Tips*:
○ Care should be exercised in determining the anatomy of the deformed cartilage. Careful dissection along the septum is important. The septum is frequently warped in any of one or more planes. Straight dissection posteriorly or inferiorly can result in perforation.

○ An idea of the shape of the septum preoperatively will help minimize the incidence of inadvertent perforation.

○ In attempting to traverse the septal cartilage but leave the contralateral septal mucosa intact, a gloved finger may be placed along the septum opposite the incision and used to palpate the depth of the knife blade. The blade should pass through only the cartilage and not the contralateral mucosa as indicated by palpation of the knife and mobility of the boundaries of the cartilage.

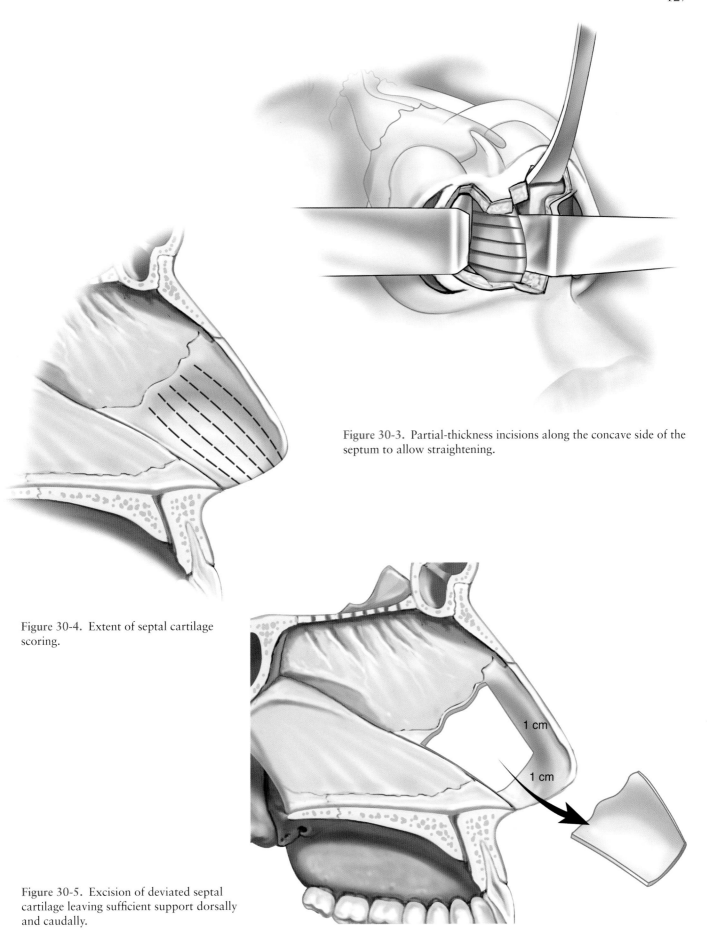

Figure 30-3. Partial-thickness incisions along the concave side of the septum to allow straightening.

Figure 30-4. Extent of septal cartilage scoring.

1 cm

1 cm

Figure 30-5. Excision of deviated septal cartilage leaving sufficient support dorsally and caudally.

Chapter 31. Turbinate Modification

- *Indications*: The turbinates should be examined at the time of the initial examination and then at each subsequent visit in addition to the day of surgery to note any changes in size and character. The three paired turbinates regulate flow (primarily the inferior) and humidify (primarily the middle) air within the nose (Figures 31-1 and 31-2). The meatuses that open near the turbinates drain the paranasal sinuses. Hypertrophy of the turbinates may interfere with normal nasal respiration. Chronic irritation and swelling acts in the nose as it does elsewhere in the body. A pattern of edema formation, gland enlargement, and fibrosis leads to hypertrophy of the underlying bone. The lifetime risk of eventual turbinate dysfunction approaches 100% as a person ages, whereas progression to persistent bothersome dysfunction is estimated to be 50%.[1]

- Etiologies of turbinate dysfunction are broad and numerous, including infections, allergies, and/or medications. Management is appropriate when clinical manifestations of turbinate pathology exist. A trial of medical management with steroid and/or antihistamine nasal sprays is a reasonable initial step and should be questioned. Often, this approach is successful for a finite period of time but then is less successful. In the instance of medication failure or contraindication, inferior turbinectomy for persistent hypertrophy of bone, mucosa, or both may be indicated. In the patient with concomitant septal deviation, replacing the septum in the midline where it now abuts a hypertrophied turbinate, may produce obstruction that was either present only on the contralateral side or nonexistent. The hypertrophy itself may also interfere with septal repositioning. Preoperatively, examination of the turbinates, especially the inferior turbinate, which is the easiest to visualize, should be performed with a nasal speculum and an adequate light source. Evidence of excessive hypertrophy should be documented.

- *Markings*: No external markings are required.

- *Approach*: Multiple techniques have been employed to address symptomatic turbinate dysfunction.
  - Cauterization with electrical current or cryotherapy with a cold agent have both been described to shrink the nasal mucosa overlying the enlarged turbinate. This may be as easy as applying the tip of the cautery into the turbinate mucosa and allowing the mucosa to coagulate. Newer techniques utilizing one of various lasers may produce less bleeding but may similarly result in recurrence of the hypertrophy.

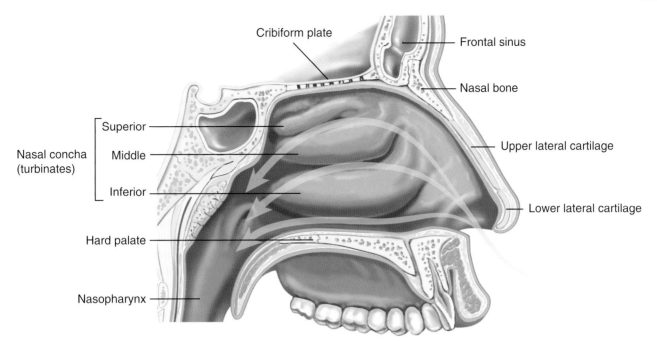

Figure 31-1. Pattern of nasal airflow across the turbinates.

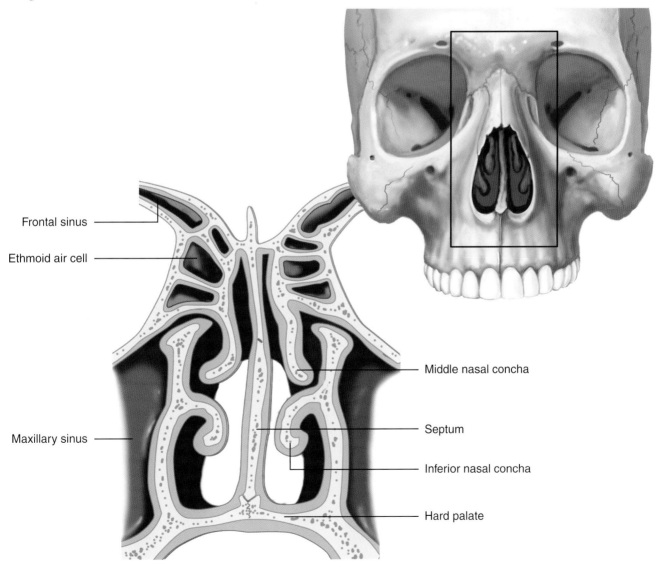

Figure 31-2. Cross-section through the nasal cavity highlighting the positions of the turbinates.

◦ For mild to moderate hypertrophy, the turbinate may be outfractured away from the septum if the hypertrophy will interfere with septal repositioning (Figure 31-3). This may be combined with any of the above techniques that shrink the nasal mucosa to minimize recurrence.

◦ For more severe hypertrophy, a portion of the turbinate can be excised (Figure 31-4). To minimize drying of inspired air, a medial mucosa flap is elevated and reflected before the turbinate bone is removed so that it may be preserved and replaced. The bone is then removed with a fine rongeur after which the mucosa is laid back down over the remaining conchal bone (Figure 31-5).

◦ Some authors have proposed a combination of coblation, which uses radiofrequency energy to ablate hypertrophied tissues, in conjunction with turbinate outfracture to relieve symptoms and maximize the nasal airway patency.[2]

- *Postoperative management*: Vaseline nasal packing can be used to moisturize and promote healing of any raw surfaces. The patient should be on antibiotics to minimize the risk of toxic shock syndrome. Thereafter, saline spray may afford some relief from drying and irritation.

- *Pitfalls*:
  ◦ Lateral nasal osteotomies that impinge on the turbinates may push them too close to the septum and produce an iatrogenic obstruction.
  ◦ The turbinates are highly vascular and can produce significant bleeding.

◦ Cauterization may lead to prolonged irritation from scab formation and scab displacement leading to delayed epistaxis.

◦ Excessive destruction of turbinate mucosa, especially the middle turbinate, can lead to drying as the ability of the nasal passages to heat and humidify the air is lost.

- *Tips*:
  ◦ The area of nasal bone between the upper and lower lateral cartilages, known as Webster's triangle, should not be violated.
  ◦ Care should be taken to maintain a low-to-low or low-to-moderate path of fracture.
  ◦ Adequate measures should taken in the operating room to ensure that bleeding is controlled, including preoperative infiltration with a vasoconstrictive agent, allowing adequate time for it to work, nasal packing at the conclusion of the procedure, and keeping the patient's head elevated for a period of time postoperatively.

REFERENCES

1. Archer SM. Turbinate dysfunction. *http://www.emedicine.com*. New York, NY. 2006.
2. Wolfswinkel EM, Koshy JC, Kaufman Y, Sharabi SE, Hollier LH Jr, Edmonds JL. A modified technique for inferior turbinate reduction: The integration of coblation technology. *Plast Reconstr Surg*. 2010 Aug;126(2):489–491.

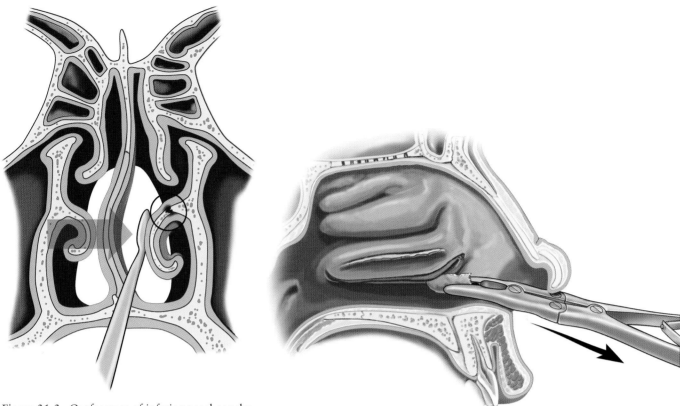

Figure 31-3. Outfracture of inferior nasal concha.

Figure 31-4. Removal of turbinate bone using a rongeur.

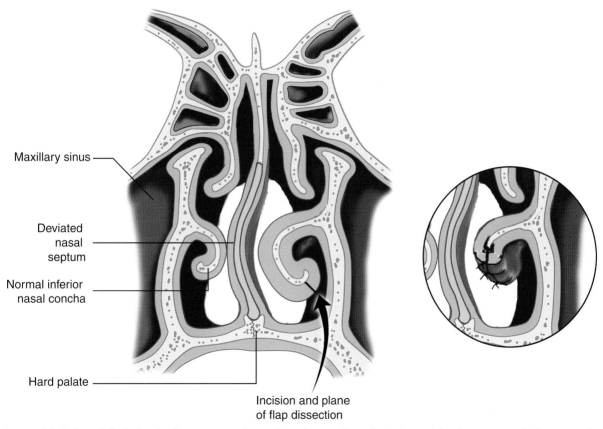

Maxillary sinus

Deviated
nasal
septum

Normal inferior
nasal concha

Hard palate

Incision and plane
of flap dissection

Figure 31-5. Septal deviation in the presence of an enlarged contralateral turbinate. After bone removal, the mucosal flap is re-sutured (inset).

Chapter 32. Closure and Dressing

- *Indications*: Following completion of the preoperatively outlined goals and objectives, the surgeon should be pleased with the result. He should not leave the operating room if there is any uncertainty of the result. If he is satisfied, a closure should be performed. Both the open and endonasal techniques of rhinoplasty require sutures to close the incisions used for access. The former requires additional sutures to close the skin and subcutaneous tissues of the columella.

- *Approach*: In general, the intranasal and external incisions are closed first, followed by placement of packing and application of an external dressing (Figure 32-1). The combination of internal packing and external splinting is commonly used to maintain the desired shape of the nose postoperatively. Internally, one or both nostrils are packed with material to provide support. Externally, the dorsum is covered with a protective splint.

- With an external approach, the subcutaneous tissues and skin of the columella should be closed with a combination of deep absorbable sutures and superficial 6-0 Prolene or nylon sutures. Many surgeons perform this two-layer closure to minimize spreading of the scar when the cuticular sutures are removed. It is important to re-create the stair-step that was made across the columella as well as the right angle transition between the horizontal and vertical portions of the columellar skin flap. Closure of the mucosal incisions may be performed with interrupted 5-0 chromic gut. If the septal mucosa was elevated to minimize hematoma formation in the potential space, 4-0 plain gut mattress sutures across the septum are recommended to eliminate the dead space.

- Nasal packing is recommended if the nasal septal mucosa was reflected. Internal nasal splints are available in silicone or a cotton material. These are removed several days after surgery. The Doyle splint actually has a hollow tube in it to facilitate nasal breathing. Some surgeons opt for nonabsorbable Vaseline gauze, which should be removed in 24 to 48 hours to improve respiration as well as minimize the incidence of infection related to the presence of a foreign body. Others opt for dissolvable cellulose packing that maintains some early support but eventually softens and is dissolved naturally. Nasal packing is often difficult to tolerate, since it forces the patient to breath through the mouth.

It is not always required and some surgeons avoid it altogether. Its use should be individualized to the patient and the procedure.

- Postoperatively, the skin over the nose has been elevated and relies on lateral perforating vessels for vascularity. Tape applied over the skin often serves two functions. It minimizes edema formation during the early postoperative period and protects the skin if the overlying splint material is too warm. Steri-strips are commonly used for this and the edges should overlap one another.

- A splint is recommended if the nasal pyramid has been manipulated. A soft splint that progressively hardens such as plaster or a thermoplastic material (Aquaplast) is preferred so that no excess pressure is placed on the osteotomized nasal bones during splint application. The stiffer aluminum splints are harder to control in terms of adapting them precisely to the new nasal dimensions, and they require more pressure to adapt to the dorsum potentially displacing nasal bones under the splint during application. If plaster is used, several layers are superimposed and then they are cut to the desired dimensions. After placing the splint in hot water (heat will set the plaster faster), it is gently applied and molded to the nose. It will warm as it hardens and can be smoothed with a moist finger while it is setting to give it a polished look. A thermoplastic splint requires very hot water. It is cut to the desired shape and size while it hardens and cools. It is then placed in hot water and transitions in color from opaque to clear as it softens. These splints are very sticky when they are soft. A nice trick is to place the splint on a gauze and then lower the gauze in the water. When the splint turns clear, the gauze can be lifted out carrying the splint to the patient for application. Both plaster and Aquaplast splints can be secured with cut Tegaderm dressings for a neat adherent dressing that is minimally cumbersome.

- *Postoperative care*: Patient's should be instructed to sleep with their head elevated. Gentle ice packs may be used in the first 24 to 48 hours to minimize swelling. While nasal breathing is certainly allowed, forceful nose blowing should be avoided. A saline mist may be used once the nasal packing has been removed to soften any residual blood or mucus to facilitate removal.

- *Tips*:
  - If nasal packing is necessary, the Doyle splint has a breathing tube in it to minimize nasal obstruction.

- Place the thermoplastic splint on a gauze and then lower the gauze in the water. The gauze can be used to move the sticky splint from water to patient minimizing handling with gloves.

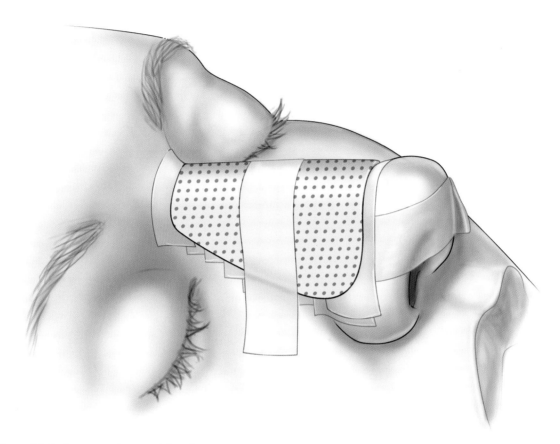

Figure 32-1. Postoperative nasal dressing.

Chapter 33. Patient Education and Consent

It should go without saying that patients undergoing rhinoplasty should be cognizant of the nature, benefits, and risks of the procedure. They should also be aware of the timeline for healing and the need to wait a minimum of 1 year before deciding that a reoperation is required. The surgeon should understand the patient's specific anatomy and particular concerns. These should be valid and consistent. The risks of each component of the planned operation should be reviewed with the patient in detail. Drawings are frequently helpful for the patient to understand the finer technicalities and to serve as a record of the detailed interaction. Preoperative photographs in standard AP, oblique, lateral, and worm's eye views should be obtained. These should also be reviewed with the patient. Software can also be used to manipulate digital images in order to provide the patient with an example of the postsurgical result. A standard consent might have similar elements to the example given below:

INFORMED CONSENT— RHINOPLASTY SURGERY

INSTRUCTIONS

The following document is an informed-consent form that has been prepared to help your plastic surgeon inform you about the nature, benefits, risks, and alternatives to rhinoplasty surgery. It is important that you read this information carefully and completely. Each page should be initialed to indicate that you have read the page and sign the consent for surgery as proposed by your surgeon.

INTRODUCTION

Rhinoplasty surgery is designed and performed to reshape or improve the function of the nose. The techniques utilized may produce changes in the appearance, structure, and function of the nose. They may reduce or increase the size of the nose or change the shape of the various components of the nose, including—but not limited to—the dorsum, tip, and nostrils. They may also change the relationship of the nose to surrounding structures, including—but not limited to—the cheeks, the eyes, and the upper lip. Rhinoplasty may be indicated to correct congenital birth defects, acquired deformities, traumatic injuries, and/or functional problems with breathing. The techniques of rhinoplasty are customized for each patient and are not identical in all patients. The techniques may be performed using either incisions outside the nose or inside the nose, or a combination of the two. Patients interested in undergoing a rhinoplasty procedure should have realistic expectations and not expect perfection. They should also be in good physical and emotional health. Rhinoplasty can be performed in conjunction with other surgeries.

RISK OF RHINOPLASTY SURGERY

With any type of surgery there is inherent risk. It is always an option not to undergo the rhinoplasty surgery. An individual's choice to undergo any particular surgical procedure is based on the comparison of the risks and potential benefit. Although the majority of patients do not experience these complications, you should discuss each of them with your plastic surgeon to make sure you understand the risks, potential complications, and consequences of rhinoplasty. Infrequently, it is necessary to perform additional surgery to improve your result.

- Bleeding—It is possible, though unusual, that you may have problem with bleeding during or after surgery. Should postoperative bleeding occur, it may require emergency treatment to stop the bleeding, or require a blood transfusion. Do not take any aspirin or antiinflammatory medications for 2 weeks before surgery, as this contributes to a greater risk of bleeding. Hypertension (high blood pressure) that is not under good medical control may cause bleeding during or after surgery. Accumulations of blood under the skin may delay healing and cause scarring.
- Infection—Infection following rhinoplasty is rare. Management usually involves a course of antibiotic therapy but may also necessitate a return to the

134

operating room for irrigation and/or debridement of infected tissue.

- Scarring—Although good wound healing after a surgical procedure is expected, abnormal scars may occur both within the skin and the deeper tissues. Scars may be unattractive and of different color than the surrounding skin. There is the possibility of visible marks from sutures. Additional treatments including surgery may be needed to treat scarring.
- Damage to deeper structures—Deeper structures such as nerves, tear ducts, blood vessels, and muscles may be damaged during the course of surgery. The potential for this to occur varies with the type of rhinoplasty procedure performed. Injury to deeper structures may be temporary or permanent.
- Nasal septal perforation—There is the possibility that surgery will cause a hole in the nasal septum to develop. This occurrence is rare. However, if it occurs, additional surgical treatment may be necessary to repair the hole in the nasal septum. In some cases, it may be impossible to correct this complication.
- Unsatisfactory result—There is the possibility of an unsatisfactory result from the rhinoplasty surgery. The surgery may result in unacceptable visible or tactile deformities, loss of function, or structural malposition after rhinoplasty surgery. You may be disappointed that the results of rhinoplasty surgery do not meet your expectations. Additional surgery may be necessary should the desired result of rhinoplasty not persist after surgery.
- Numbness—There is the potential for permanent numbness within the nasal skin after rhinoplasty. The occurrence of this is not predictable. Diminished (or loss of skin sensation) in the nasal area may not totally resolve rhinoplasty.
- Asymmetry—The human face is normally asymmetrical. There can be a variation from one side to the other in the results obtained from a rhinoplasty procedure.
- Chronic pain—Chronic pain may occur very infrequently after rhinoplasty.
- Allergic reactions—In rare cases, local allergies to tape, suture material, or topical preparations have been reported. Systemic reactions, which are more serious, may occur to drugs used during surgery and prescription medicines. Allergic reactions may require additional treatment.
- Delayed healing—Wound disruption or delayed wound healing is possible. Some areas of the face may not heal normally and may take a long time to heal. Areas of skin may die. This may require frequent dressing changes or further surgery to remove the non-healed tissue.
- Long-term effects—Subsequent alterations in nasal appearance may occur as the result of aging, sun exposure, or other circumstances not related to rhinoplasty surgery. Future surgery or other treatments may be necessary to maintain the results of a rhinoplasty operation.

- Nasal airway alteration—Changes may occur after a rhinoplasty or septoplasty operation that may interfere with normal passage of air through the nose.
- Surgical anesthesia—Both local and general anesthesia involve risk. There is the possibility of complications, injury, and even death from all forms of surgical anesthesia or sedation.

ADDITIONAL ADVISORIES

Deep Venous Thrombosis and Pulmonary Complications: Surgery, especially longer procedures, may be associated with the formation of blood clots in the venous system. Complications may occur secondarily if blood clots (pulmonary emboli), or fat deposits (fat emboli), travel to the lungs. Pulmonary and fat emboli can be life threatening or fatal in some circumstances. Air travel, inactivity, and other conditions may increase the incidence of blood clots travelling to the lungs causing a major blood clot that may result in death. It is important to discuss with your plastic surgeon any past history of blood clots or swollen legs that may contribute to this condition.

Smoking, Second-Hand Smoke Exposure, Nicotine Products (Patch, Gum, Nasal Spray): Patients who are currently smoking, use tobacco products, or nicotine products (patch, gum, or nasal spray) are at a greater risk for significant surgical complications of skin necrosis, delayed healing, and additional scarring. Individuals exposed to second-hand smoke are also at potential risk for similar complications attributable to nicotine exposure. Additionally, smokers may have a significant negative effect on anesthesia and recovery from anesthesia, with coughing and possibly increased bleeding. It is important to refrain from smoking at least 6 weeks before surgery and until your physician states it is safe to return, if desired.

Information Specific to Female Patients: It is important to inform your plastic surgeon if you use birth control pills or estrogen replacement, or if you believe you may be pregnant. Many medications including antibiotics may neutralize the preventive effect of birth control pills, allowing for conception and pregnancy.

Medications: Numerous adverse reactions may occur as the result of taking over-the-counter and/or prescription medications and/or herbal supplements. Be sure to check with your plastic surgeon about any drug interactions that may exist with medications you are already taking. If you have an adverse reaction, stop the drugs immediately and call your plastic surgeon for further instructions. If the reaction is severe, go immediately to the nearest emergency room. When taking the prescribed pain medications after surgery, realize that they can affect your thought process. Do not drive, do not operate complex equipment, do not make any important decisions, and do not drink any alcohol while taking these medications. Be sure to take your prescribed medication only as directed.

HEALTH INSURANCE

Most insurance companies exclude coverage for cosmetic surgical operations or any complications that might occur from cosmetic surgery. If the procedure corrects a breathing problem or marked deformity after a nasal fracture, a portion may be covered. Please carefully review your health insurance subscriber policy.

FINANCIAL RESPONSIBILITIES

The total cost of surgery involves several component charges for the services provided. The total cost includes your surgeon's fee, your anesthesiologist's fee, and outpatient facility charges, as well as possible additional laboratory charges. Depending on whether the cost of surgery is covered by an insurance plan, you will be responsible for necessary co-payments, deductibles, and charges not covered. Additional costs may occur should complications develop from the surgery. Secondary surgery or hospital day surgery charges involved with revisionary surgery would also be your responsibility.

PATIENT COMPLIANCE

All instructions given by your physician should be carefully followed to maximize the success of your outcome. It is important that the surgical incisions are not subjected to excessive force, swelling, abrasion, or motion during the time of healing. Physical activity needs to be restricted. Surgery involves clotting of blood vessels and increased activity of any kind may open these vessels, leading to a bleed, or hematoma. Increased activity that raises your pulse or heart rate may cause additional bruising, swelling, and the need for return to surgery and control of bleeding. It is wise to refrain from physical exertion (including sexual activity) until your physician determines it is safe. Protective dressings and drains should not be removed unless instructed by your plastic surgeon. Successful postoperative function depends on both surgery and subsequent care. It is important that you participate in follow-up care, return for aftercare, and promote your recovery after surgery.

DISCLAIMER

Informed-consent documents are used to communicate information about the proposed surgical treatment of a disease or condition along with disclosure of risks and alternative forms of treatment(s). This documents is based on a thorough evaluation of scientific literature and relevant clinic practice to describe a range of generally acceptable risks and alternative forms of management of a particular disease or condition. The informed-consent process attempts to define principles of risk disclosure that should generally meet the needs of most patients in most circumstances. However, informed-consent documents should not be considered all inclusive in defining other methods of care and risks encountered. Your plastic surgeon may provide you with additional or different information that is based on all the facts in your particular case and the state of medical knowledge. Informed-consent documents are not intended to define or serve as the standard of medical care. Standards of medical care are determined on the basis of all of the facts involved in an individual case and are subject to change as scientific knowledge and technology advance and as practice patterns evolve. This informed-consent document reflects the state of knowledge current at the time of publication. It is important that you have read the above information carefully and have all of your questions answered before signing the consent.

Chapter 34. Coding

Jay Meisner, MD, FACS

- **Brief History:** The fourth edition of *Current Procedural Terminology* (CPT, 2011 modification)[1] was developed by the American Medical Association (AMA) and was published for first use in 1966. Its initial purpose was unrelated to reimbursement; it was developed as a type of medical shorthand for documenting and recording procedures. In 1983, the Health Care Financial Administration (HCFA) mandated that CPT be used as a standardized method for Medicare billing. This was extended to include Medicaid billing in 1986. Major insurers soon began to mandate its use, and would reject any medical claims not using CPT coding.[2]

- **Purpose of CPT coding:** Today, CPT coding is a standardized means by which a medical provider most accurately describes procedures performed. It may be used as a tool for documentation alone, as with purely aesthetic procedures. More commonly, it must be used as a communication tool to health insurers to accurately document procedures performed and to obtain appropriate reimbursement.

- The **International classification of diseases**[3] (ICD) originated in seventeenth-century England, and its current ninth revision (ICD-9) is used to describe medical diagnoses. Using the most specific ICD-9 code(s) matching the specific CPT code(s) of the procedures (to be) performed is the best way to communicate what was done, and for what reason. Insurers will deny payment for viable claims if the ICD-9 code does not match the CPT code.
  - *Cosmetic vs. reconstructive surgery*: In 1989, the AMA adopted the following definitions of cosmetic and reconstructive surgery, which is reiterated in the American Society of Plastic Surgeons (ASPS) Recommended Insurance Coverage Criteria for Third-Party Payers. *Cosmetic* surgery is performed to reshape normal structures of the body in order to improve the patient's appearance and self-esteem. *Reconstructive* surgery is performed on abnormal structures of the body, caused by congenital defects, developmental abnormalities, trauma, infection, tumors, or disease. It is generally performed to improve function, but may also be done to approximate a normal appearance.[4]

  - The treating physician must carefully assess the potential patient to determine whether the proposed procedure is purely elective and aesthetic, purely reconstructive, or a combination of cosmetic and reconstructive procedures.
  - *Combined cosmetic and reconstructive procedures*: When rhinoplasty has both cosmetic and functional components, it is always important to preauthorize the procedures in writing, to be sure to distinguish which components are reconstructive (both preoperatively and in a single operative dictation), and to not bill the carrier for the cosmetic components.[5] It is worthwhile to quote the AMA definitions above in the preauthorization request. Similarly, it is recommended that the cosmetic and reconstructive portions are clearly itemized for the patient in writing. The patient should understand the cost of the cosmetic component as well as any deductibles, coinsurances, and balances above and beyond the usual and customary reimbursement for the reconstructive portion.

- **Elective aesthetic rhinoplasty:** CPT coding for elective, purely aesthetic rhinoplasty may be used for documentation of the type and extent of the procedure for the physician's medical records. Practices may use and analyze this documentation for practice management, procedure trends, combined procedure analysis, and marketing. Although not mandated, the use of aesthetic rhinoplasty codes in combination with functional CPT codes may serve to fully document which portions of a combined procedure are aesthetic and non-reimbursable and which portions are functional and reimbursable.
  - When ICD-9 coding is necessary, V50.1 (plastic surgery for unacceptable cosmetic appearance) may be used.
  - CPT codes may be used to document the various types and extent of aesthetic rhinoplasty. Primary rhinoplasty implies no prior nasal surgery. Secondary rhinoplasty implies prior nasal surgery by the treating surgeon or by another surgeon.

- **Reconstructive rhinoplasty and related procedures:** It is imperative that any and all proposed reconstructive rhinoplasty and related procedures be preauthorized by the involved health insurance carrier *in writing* prior to performing such procedures. CPT codes for rhinoplasty do not and cannot directly indicate whether the procedure is cosmetic or reconstructive. Most rhinoplasty CPT codes may be construed as cosmetic in nature, so complete documentation of the reconstructive nature of the proposed procedures must be conveyed to the carrier and acknowledged as reimbursable. Both primary and secondary rhinoplasty codes not only describe procedures performed electively for correction of primary nasal deformities and post-rhinoplasty deformities, respectively, but they may be used to report treatment of an array of functional and/or reconstructive nasal problems. In the event that any of the above procedures are performed for functional reasons, appropriate pre-procedure authorization as well as post-procedure documentation of the extent and nature of the procedure performed must accompany any insurance billing.

- The following ICD-9 codes, which are not meant to be fully inclusive, may be used to describe the most common functional problems in reconstructive rhinoplasty (Table 34-1):

- **CPT Coding of reconstructive rhinoplasty procedures:** The following is a listing of the most common reconstructive rhinoplasty codes. It is imperative to match the diagnosis code(s) with the CPT code(s) and to document all procedures performed in detail in the operative report. There is no distinction made as to the surgical approach, whether open or endonasal (Table 34-2).

- The following graft codes may be used in addition to the primary procedure codes (Table 34-3):

- **Coding of traumatic nasal fractures and their sequelae:** Acute traumatic nasal fractures (closed, ICD-9 802.0 or open, ICD-9 802.1) are often treated by closed reduction with or without stabilization (CPT 21315 or 21320). The results of closed reduction, however, may not be optimal and may require a secondary procedure to restore the nose to the pre-injury

state. If the fracture is healed, it is no longer an acute fracture and using 21315 or 21320 again is not indicated. The use of a primary rhinoplasty code is appropriate, yet if only osteotomies are performed, there is no appropriate primary rhinoplasty CPT code. Therefore, CPT 30410-52 may be used, indicating the bony work was performed without the cartilage work. Of course, appropriate detailed documentation is required.[6]

- **The use of CPT modifiers:** CPT modifiers may be used to denote services above and beyond the usual magnitude of the procedure (-22) or diminished services (-52). These modifiers serve to increase or diminish services not sufficiently described by the particular CPT code.

  - The postoperative period, when any additional procedures are considered incidental to the primary procedure, is usually 90 days. Staged procedures performed within this postoperative period may be identified using the -58 modifier. An unplanned return to the operating room during the postoperative period must be billed with the -78 modifier. An unrelated procedure (eg, removal of a skin cancer during the postoperative period for a submucous resection) must be billed with a -79 modifier.

  - Bilateral procedures are denoted by the -50 modifier. Some carriers prefer the use of –LT and –RT.

  - Although the -51 modifier may be used to denote multiple procedures (using -51 for any procedures after the first), omitting it rarely has any effect on claims processing.

- **Unbundling of procedures:** When a single CPT code exists that describes a combination of procedures, it is not appropriate to separately bill each part of the procedure with an individual code. In many cases, the CPT manual makes note of codes not usable with certain other codes. This unbundling of procedure codes is usually picked up at the initial claims processing level, when sophisticated claims processing algorithms deny codes, which are documented as being a part of another procedure. This may occur even in the face of a fully preauthorized listing of CPT codes. For example, CPT 30420 (complete rhinoplasty with major septal repair) includes CPT 30520 (septoplasty or submucous resection).

  - It is recommended that any and all proposed procedure codes be carefully reviewed for inclusive components prior to preauthorization or billing. Of course, if there is a denial of a code that is felt to not be bundled into another code, the claim should be appealed with a detailed explanation.

- **Criteria for insurance coverage for reconstructive rhinoplasty and related procedures:** Many third-party payers (health insurers) have specific criteria that need to be met prior to approving proposed reconstructive

Table 34-1

ICD-9	Description
095.5	Saddle nose deformity
470.0	Deviated nasal septum, acquired
478.0	Nasal turbinate hypertrophy
478.1	Nasal airway obstruction
709.2	Scar
733.81	Malunion of nasal/septal fracture
748.1	Congenital nasal deformity
754.0	Congenital nasal/septal deformity
905.0	Late effect of fracture of skull or facial bones

Table 34-2

CPT	Procedure (Reconstructive Rhinoplasty)	Comments
30400	Primary rhinoplasty: lateral and alar cartilages and/or tip	May be used for congenital, traumatic, or extirpative soft tissue deformities. This codes rhinoplasty without bony work.
30410	Primary rhinoplasty: lateral and alar cartilages, tip, bony pyramid	May be used to code correction of soft tissue deformities with osteotomies. It may also code osteotomy only without a tip or cartilage procedure, using the -52 modifier. This codes rhinoplasty with osteotomies. It may also code osteotomy only without a tip or cartilage procedure, adding the -52 modifier.
30420	Primary rhinoplasty: lateral and alar cartilages, tip, bony pyramid, including major septal repair	Use this code when performing reconstructive rhinoplasty in conjunction with septal work. Use 30520 for isolated septal work. Septal repair may be done for nonfunctional reasons such as non-obstructive deformity or caudal dislocation.
30430	Secondary rhinoplasty: minor revision, nasal tip	Be sure to document the indications for functional tip revision. Note that the secondary codes are somewhat different from the primary codes.
30435	Secondary rhinoplasty: bony work with osteotomies	This code is best used for correction of secondary bony deformities.
30450	Secondary rhinoplasty: nasal tip and osteotomies	
30520	Septoplasty or submucous resection	Use this code alone or in addition to a secondary reconstructive rhinoplasty code. There is no CPT code for isolated septal work during a secondary rhinoplasty. This code may also be used for primary nonfunctional septoplasty.
30130	Excision inferior turbinate, partial or complete, any method	Note that turbinate codes are by default bilateral.
30140	Submucous resection inferior turbinate, partial or complete, any method	Use -52 modifier for "reduction" of turbinates (eg, needle cautery)
30460	Cleft lip rhinoplasty including columellar lengthening; tip work only	Columellar lengthening is included in 30460 and 30462.
30462	Cleft lip rhinoplasty; tip, septum, osteotomies	This code contains all soft tissue and bony components. May use -52 modifier if only bony work is done. May be used in addition to the cleft lip nose repair codes 30460 or 30462.
30465	Repair vestibular stenosis (spreader grafting, lateral nasal wall reconstruction)	Be sure to add the appropriate code for the graft used (below).

rhinoplasty procedures. These criteria may usually be found at the carrier's website or by request. By obtaining a specific insurer's criteria, steps toward preauthorization may be optimized.

○ The most common indications for nasal reconstructive surgery include impaired nasal respiratory function (including decreased or altered airway flow), anatomic abnormalities caused by birth defects or disease, or structural deformities due to trauma. Congenital deformities, such as cleft lip nasal deformity or developmental anomalies may be covered even if there is no functional deficit; often the carrier denies the preauthorization request if no true functional deficit exists. It requires diligence and persistence, and on occasion a peer-to-peer discussion with a medical director, to convince the carrier that the patient has a congenital deformity requiring correction in order to approximate a normal appearance.[2]

• **Methods of documentation for preauthorization:** The treating surgeon should accurately document the patient's pertinent medical history, past surgical history, social history, and detailed physical examination findings. A written referral from the referring provider

Table 34-3

CPT	Procedure (Additional or Ancillary Procedures)	Comments
15760	Graft, composite	
20912	Septal cartilage graft to nose	May not be used with 30420, 30462 or 30520, as these are primary septal codes.
20926	Tissue grafts, other (paratenon, fat, dermis)	
21210	Bone graft to nose (includes obtaining graft)	
21230	Rib cartilage graft to nose (includes obtaining graft)	
21235	Ear cartilage graft to nose (includes obtaining graft)	

may help to strengthen the indications for surgery. Reports from other treating physicians as well as any prior operative reports or photographs should be obtained. Preoperative photographs, as indicated, should be clearly labeled with the patient's name, the surgeon's name, and the date taken.

- ○ Any and all functional abnormalities and/or nasal defects should be documented, not limited to: visible or palpable deformities, visible degree of septal deviation, degree of turbinate hypertrophy, difficulty breathing at rest and with exercise, effect of external nasal repositioning on airflow (Cottle maneuver).
- ○ For congenital anomalies or traumatic injuries, it is important to document the significance of how it deviates from the norm, and in some cases how it impacts the individual psychosocially.
- ○ Diagnostic studies may be performed as clinically indicated, including facial X-rays, CT or MRI scans, nasal endoscopy, and/or nasal airflow studies.
- ○ When submitting a written preauthorization request, include as much pertinent documentation as possible, trying to meet all of the specific carrier's criteria. It is worthwhile requesting that a board-certified plastic surgeon review the preauthorization request.
- ○ Some practices send preauthorization requests via traceable mail carrier. It is recommended the carrier be called to confirm receipt and to follow up the request in timely fashion.
- ○ Obtaining preauthorization *in writing* is strongly recommended prior to performing surgery.
- **Handling preauthorization denials:** Denials for preauthorization should be received in writing. Many carriers

do not give detailed explanations, and often the request is reviewed by a clerk or nurse. Unless the carrier specifically excludes the proposed procedure(s), it is worthwhile to appeal their decision in writing and, if possible, with a peer-to-peer discussion with the individual who denied the request. Denial by a non-physician should be followed by an immediate request that a physician (preferably a board-certified plastic surgeon) review the request.

- ○ Despite clear indications and documentation, many preauthorization requests are denied. The surgeon and staff should follow all appeal procedures in the hope that escalating the exposure to higher ranking carrier's representatives and medical directors will lead to preauthorization of indicated procedures.
- ○ Persistent denials for these types of procedures may require involvement of the local Medical Society's insurance advocate. If the coverage is not a self-funded plan, an external appeal with the state's Department of Insurance may be possible.
- ○ Finally, it may be advantageous to involve the patient in the process. Depending on the nature of the anomaly or deformity, a personal appeal by the patient to the carrier may have positive results.
- **Billing of reconstructive rhinoplasty procedure:** A carefully itemized billing should include the following:
  - ○ Standard HCFA billing form with appropriate CPT codes and modifiers
  - ○ Matching ICD-9 diagnosis codes
  - ○ Appropriate modifiers
  - ○ Preauthorization reference number
  - ○ A copy of the written preauthorization
  - ○ The operative report, which should clearly make note of the patient's history, symptoms, physical findings, prior surgery, and specific indications for surgery. "All proposed procedures have been preauthorized in writing by the carrier" may be added.
- **Medicare billing:** There are several situations that distinguish the billing of procedures for Medicare beneficiaries. There is no preauthorization necessary or possible with Medicare. Documentation or operative reports may not be sent in with Medicare billings. As most rhinoplasty codes may represent either aesthetic or reconstructive procedures, documentation is paramount. Many functional rhinoplasty procedures are summarily denied and must be appealed. In the case of a Medicare patient who will undergo either a purely elective nasal procedure, or where a portion is considered cosmetic, it is imperative that patient understand and sign a Medicare Advance Beneficiary Notice of Non-Coverage.[7] This informs the patient that part or all of their surgery will not be covered by Medicare.

REFERENCES

1. *Current Procedural Terminology.* 4th ed., 2011 Modification. American Medical Association; 2011.
2. *Taubman S. Medical Laboratory Observer.* October 2000.
3. *International Classification of Diseases.* 9th ed., Clinical Modification (ICD-9-CM). 2011.
4. American Society of Plastic Surgeons. *Recommended Insurance Coverage Criteria for Third-Party Payers: Nasal Surgery.* July 2006.
5. Janevicius, R. CPT corner: Cosmetic or reconstructive rhinoplasty? *Plastic Surgery News.* May 1995.
6. Documentation Critical When Billing for Late Repair of Nasal Fractures. supercoder.com. May 2000.
7. Medicare Advance Beneficiary Notice of Non-Coverage. www.cms.gov/MLNProducts/downloads/ABN_Booklet_ICN006266.pdf

Appendix

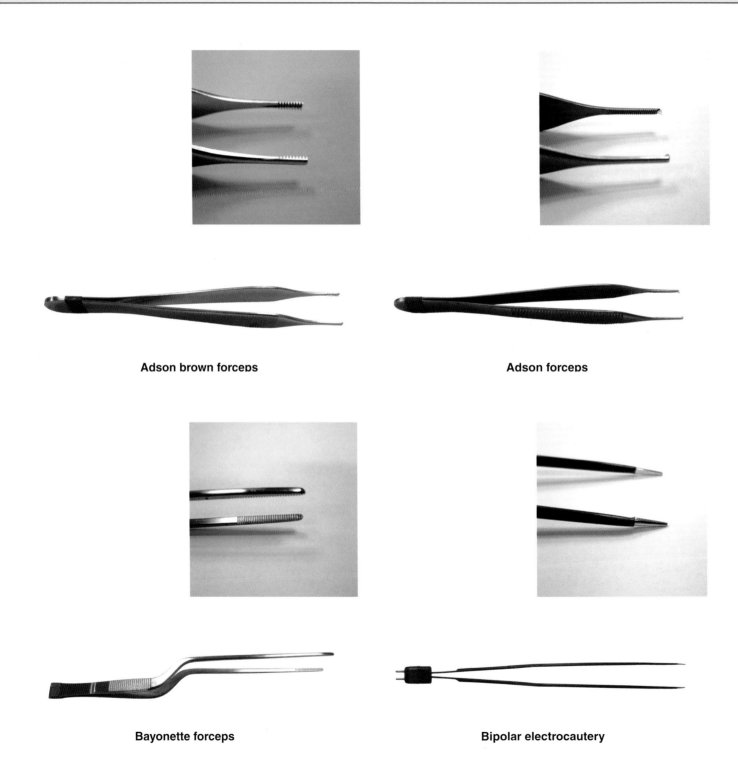

Adson brown forceps

Adson forceps

Bayonette forceps

Bipolar electrocautery

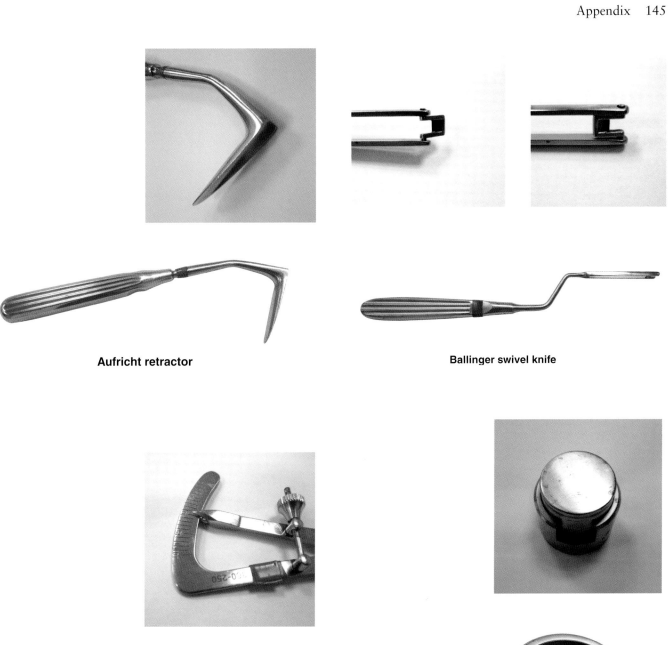

Aufricht retractor

Ballinger swivel knife

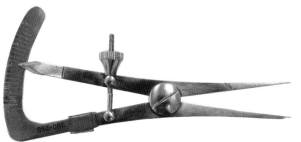

Calipers

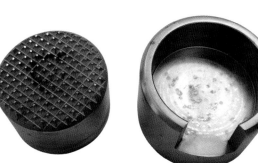

Cartilage crusher

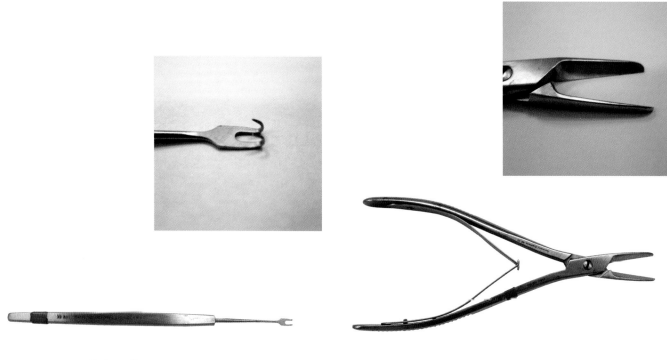

Columellar retractor

Cottle nasal scissors

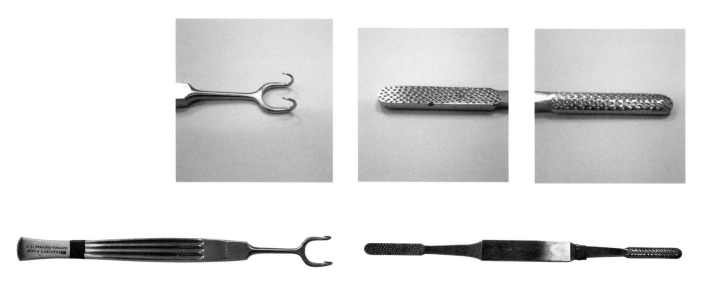

Double hook retractor

Double-sided nasal rasp

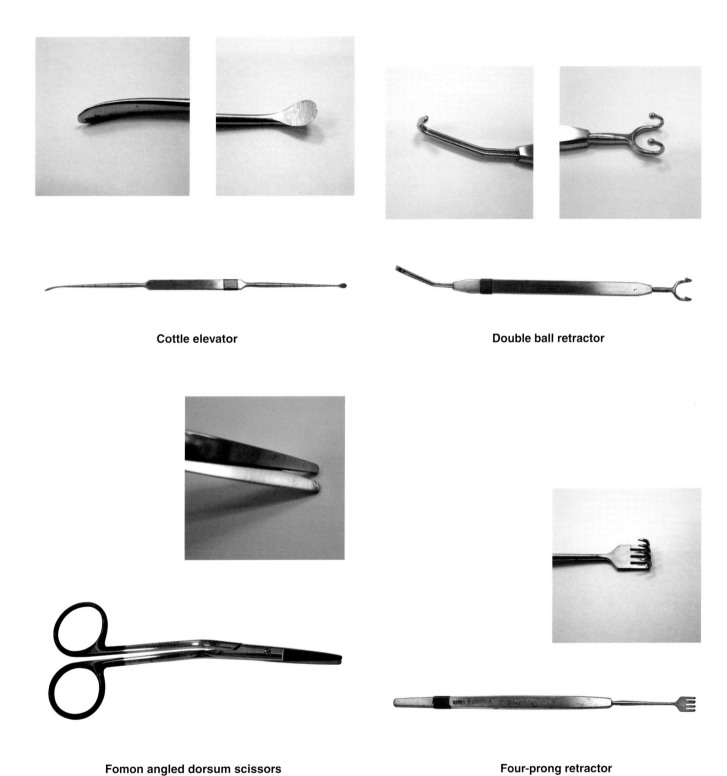

Cottle elevator

Double ball retractor

Fomon angled dorsum scissors

Four-prong retractor

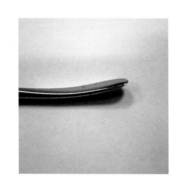

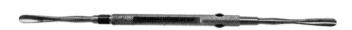

Freer elevator

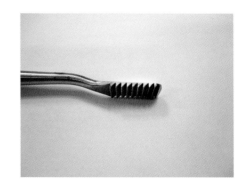

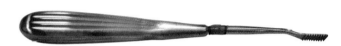

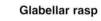

Glabellar rasp

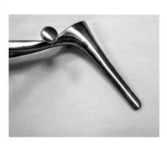

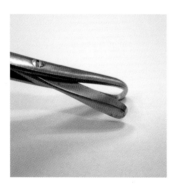

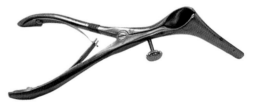

Long nasal speculum

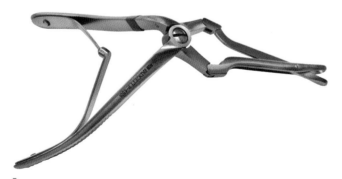

Jansen-Middleton through-action forceps

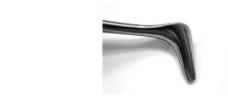

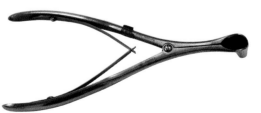

Short nasal speculum

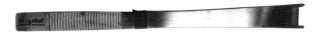

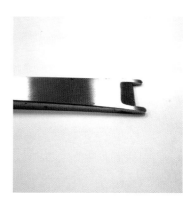

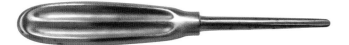

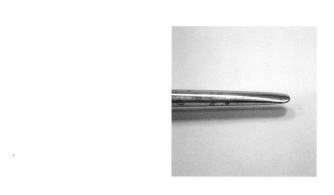

Goldman elevator

Straight guarded osteotome

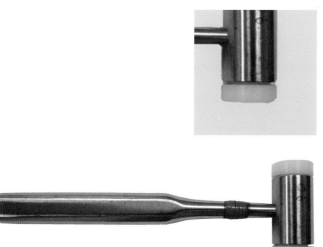

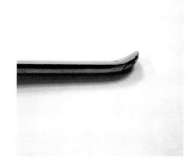

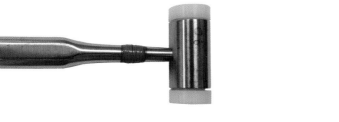

Osteotomy mallet

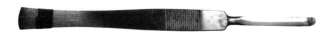

McKenty septal periosteal elevator

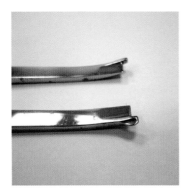

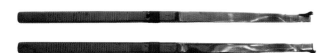

Curved nasal osteotomes

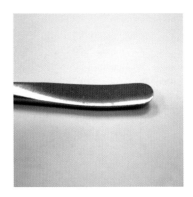

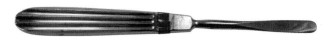

Obwegeser periosteal elevator

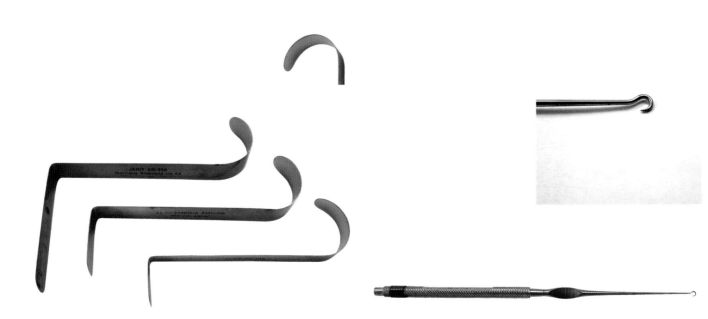

Septal (Ribbon) retractors

Single hook retractor

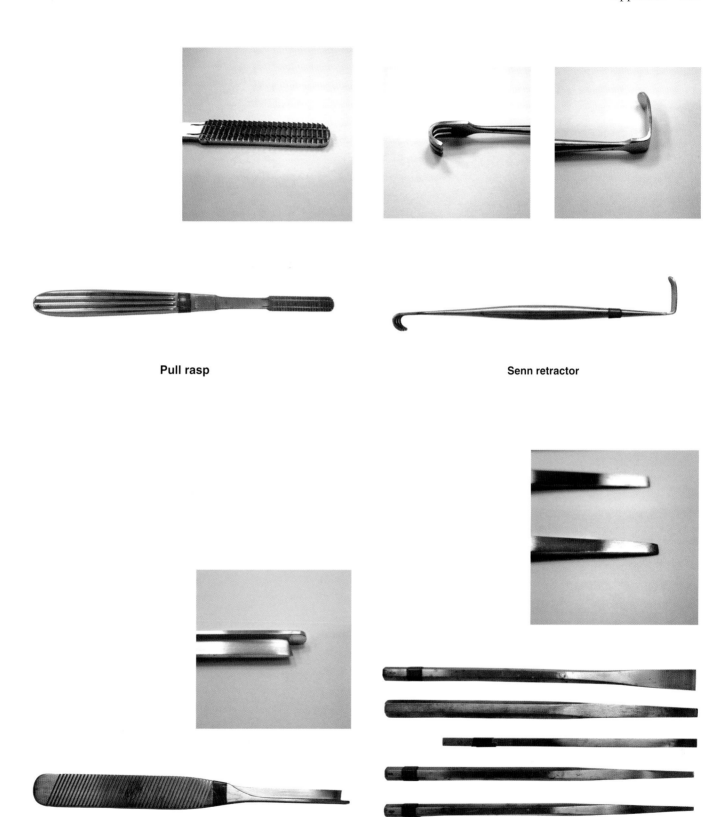

Pull rasp

Senn retractor

Straight nasal osteotome

Straight osteotomes

Index

Page numbers followed by *f* and *t* indicate figures and tables, respectively.